# Praise for *Androgen Deprivation Therapy*

"It was only when I began my personal journey with androgen deprivation therapy (ADT) that I was able to appreciate the profound impact this treatment has on daily life. Even with my real-life experience with ADT, accumulated over a decade, I know I cannot, within limits of one or even several office visits, begin to prepare and educate patients for their new reality. I could not even do that for myself! If only a complete user-friendly manual existed. Now it does."

—Paul F. Schellhammer, MD, Eastern Virginia Medical School/
Urology of Virginia and past president of the American Urological Association

"Androgen deprivation therapy (ADT) is a life-changing event, leaving many men feeling as if they have washed-up on a deserted island with no one to talk to. And that is largely true, because unless a person has been through it, and most doctors have not, it is impossible to understand how the patient feels and how to help. And for their wives, it can be like having a stranger in their bed. Until now, there has been no convenient source for patients and their physicians to get the answers that they need. However, with the publication of *Androgen Deprivation Therapy*, at last there is a comprehensive book that covers everything: side effects, diet, exercise, psychological issues, and sexual relations. And beyond helping patients understand what is going on with their body, there is encouragement and there are concrete, practical exercises and solutions. Every man who is a candidate for ADT needs to read this outstanding book."

— Patrick C. Walsh, MD, University Distinguished Service Professor of Urology,
The Johns Hopkins Medical Institutions

"A fantastic, pragmatic, well-written book. Very comprehensive."

—Derek R. Wilke, MD, Department of Radiation Oncology,
Nova Scotia Cancer Centre

"This book is an incredibly valuable resource for men with prostate cancer considering androgen deprivation therapy (ADT) and for their families and friends. It will help men to understand the pros and cons of ADT treatment and give them an idea of what to expect after they start therapy. I will certainly use it in my practice and encourage other physicians to do so as well."

—David F. Penson, MD, MPH, Hamilton and Howd Chair in Urologic Oncology,
Professor of Urologic Surgery and Medicine, Director, Center for Surgical Quality and
Outcomes Research, Vanderbilt University Medical Center

"Excellent, very informative, and comprehensive. *Androgen Deprivation Therapy* addresses issues sensitively, and is not afraid to tackle important but often ignored topics. I would be glad to recommend it to my patients."

—Paul D. Abel, ChM, FRCS (Eng), FRCS (Ed), Professor and Honorary Consultant in
Urology, Imperial College London

# ANDROGEN DEPRIVATION THERAPY

# ANDROGEN DEPRIVATION THERAPY

## AN ESSENTIAL GUIDE FOR PROSTATE CANCER PATIENTS AND THEIR LOVED ONES

**Richard J. Wassersug, PhD**
**Lauren M. Walker, PhD**
**John W. Robinson, PhD, R Psych**

*with Contributions from*
Kristen L. Currie, MA, CCRP; Kirsten Kukula, BSc;
Linette Lawlor-Savage, MSc; Andrew Matthew, PhD, C Psych;
Deborah McLeod, RN, PhD; Daniel Santa Mina, CEP, PhD;
Cheri Van Patten, RD, MSc

Reviewed and endorsed by the Canadian Urological Association,
August 2013.

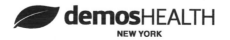

**demos**HEALTH

**NEW YORK**

Visit our website at www.demoshealth.com

*ISBN:* 978-1-936303-66-3
*e-book ISBN:* 978-1-617052-20-0

*Acquisitions Editor:* Julia Pastore
*Compositor:* diacriTech

Medical information provided by Demos Health, in the absence of a visit with a health care professional, must be considered as an educational service only. This book is not designed to replace a physician's independent judgment about the appropriateness or risks of a procedure or therapy for a given patient. Our purpose is to provide you with information that will help you make your own health care decisions.

The information and opinions provided here are believed to be accurate and sound, based on the best judgment available to the authors, editors, and publisher, but readers who fail to consult appropriate health authorities assume the risk of injuries. The publisher is not responsible for errors or omissions. The editors and publisher welcome any reader to report to the publisher any discrepancies or inaccuracies noticed.

**Library of Congress Cataloging-in-Publication Data**

Wassersug, Richard J. (Richard Joel), 1946- author.
   Androgen deprivation therapy : an essential guide for prostate cancer patients and their loved ones / Richard J. Wassersug, PhD, Lauren M. Walker, PhD, John W. Robinson, PhD, RPsych ; with contribution from Kristen L. Currie, MA, CCRP [and 6 others].
      pages cm
   "Reviewed and endorsed by the Canadian Urological Association, August 2013."
   Includes bibliographical references and index.
   ISBN 978-1-936303-66-3—ISBN 978-1-61705-220-0 (e-book)
1. Prostate—Cancer—Hormone therapy. 2. Antiandrogens—Therapeutic use. 3. Prostate—Cancer—Popular works. I. Walker, Lauren M. (Lauren Marie), 1985- author. II. Robinson, John W. (John Wellesley), 1956- author. III. Title.
   RC280.P7W37 2014
   616.99'463—dc23
                                        2014010835

Special discounts on bulk quantities of Demos Health books are available to corporations, professional associations, pharmaceutical companies, health care organizations, and other qualifying groups. For details, please contact:

Special Sales Department
Demos Medical Publishing, LLC
11 West 42nd Street, 15th Floor
New York, NY 10036
Phone: 800-532-8663 or 212-683-0072
Fax: 212-941-7842
E-mail: specialsales@demosmedical.com

Printed in the United States of America by McNaughton & Gunn.
16 17 18 / 8 7 6

*This book is dedicated to all of the men, and their partners, who have taught us what life is like on androgen deprivation therapy.*

# Contents

# Foreword

In the days before prostate-specific antigen (PSA) could be measured by a blood test, it was common for men to appear in the doctor's office complaining about pain, which would turn out to be due to the spread of prostate cancer to their bones. The standard therapy at that time was orchiectomy, or surgical removal of the testicles. The testicles produce testosterone, a male hormone, or androgen, known to stimulate the growth of prostate cancer. In the early 1940s, this procedure had been shown to relieve pain due to metastatic prostate cancer, and thus became the "gold standard" for treating the disease. The early 1980s saw the approval of injectable drugs called gonadotropin-releasing hormone (GnRH, also called luteinizing hormone-releasing hormone, LHRH) analogs, which offered a much needed alternative to the permanent orchiectomy. Since these drugs could turn off the testicular production of the androgen testosterone, the treatment was called *androgen deprivation therapy* (ADT). Many men opted for the drugs rather than orchiectomy.

Soon after the GnRH analogs became available, the U.S. Food and Drug Administration (FDA) approved the PSA test. Over time, this test allowed us to find a whole new population of prostate cancer patients, namely, those men who had had surgery or radiation for localized prostate cancer and who now had a rising PSA measurement without any evidence of disease having spread to their bones or elsewhere. This condition is commonly called "biochemical relapse" because only the blood test indicates return of the cancer. Out of concern for the continuously rising PSA, we often started ADT, even though the men did not have any evidence of metastases. In most cases, ADT was very successful in bringing the PSA down to undetectable levels for long periods of time.

However, I began to hear from patients treated with ADT shots for biochemical relapse that they were feeling fatigued and experiencing a whole host of other symptoms. In the past, I had often encountered men with metastatic disease, who had either started the ADT injections or had had an orchiectomy, complain of fatigue. My naïve response was, "Of course you have some fatigue. You have metastatic prostate cancer." But now a light bulb went off: the fatigue and other symptoms experienced by the biochemical relapse patients were from the ADT! Unlike the men I had encountered earlier in my practice, these men did not have metastases and had been feeling fine before the shots were started. Thus began an era of intense clinical research on the effects of ADT on the physiology, psychology, and cognitive functioning of men so treated.

The list of potential side effects of ADT is lengthy, and the list of different ways to address these side effects is even longer. Busy physicians may have only enough time to skim over these details, leaving the patient and his family unprepared for what to expect. In spite of our best efforts to educate patients and their partners about ADT, we often still feel we are not doing enough.

I met Richard Wassersug in 2006, when he came to Seattle for a visit. He was interested in intermittent ADT, and we met in a conference room with Monique Cherrier, PhD, my colleague who has collaborated with me in studying the effects of ADT on cognitive function. Dr. Wassersug explained that he was a scientist who primarily studied amphibian developmental biology, but, more importantly for our conversation, he was a man who had prostate cancer. As a scientist, he was a keen observer of the side effects of ADT and was also doing some laboratory and clinical research with colleagues in Halifax on the effects of ADT. Through research, personal observation, and staying in tune with men treated with ADT all over the world via Internet blogs and websites, Dr. Wassersug has accumulated a vast understanding of the side effects, how to explain them, and how to talk with men about dealing with them.

Around the same time as my meeting him, Dr. Wassersug sought out Dr. Robinson of the Tom Baker Cancer Centre. Soon they began collaborating. Dr. Robinson, a renowned psychosocial oncologist working with couples affected by cancer, clearly valued the dual perspective of Dr. Wassersug, the prostate cancer patient, and Dr. Wassersug, the research scientist.

Dr. Robinson and his then student, Lauren Walker, have since then been collaborating with Dr. Wassersug on various projects related to ADT. Dr. Wassersug found in Drs. Robinson and Walker specialized clinical skills, patient education expertise, and invaluable knowledge of a broad range of patient experiences. Equally passionate about improving the lives of men on ADT, these three individuals, plus other collaborators along the way, have significantly changed the ways in which patients are cared for while on ADT.

As a research team, Drs. Wassersug, Robinson, and Walker have found that patients and their partners remain poorly informed about the side effects of ADT. They established an ADT Working Group of about 20 professionals (i.e., researchers and clinicians) that make recommendations about the psychosocial care of men on ADT. Their research has demonstrated considerable variability in the information that health care professionals believe to be essential to provide to patients. As a team, Drs. Wassersug, Robinson, and Walker have worked to develop educational initiatives for patients, partners, and health care professionals, to help patients prepare for and manage the changes associated with ADT. This book is the culmination of several years of their work.

This book is different from consultations with specialists or conversations with nurses and doctors: it is something you can take home, read, and work on at your own pace, on your own time. You can read it in whatever order is of interest, skipping sections that may not be significant to you at this time, or going back and reviewing specific sections later. Importantly, this book emphasizes the impact of ADT on partners, so if you have one, it is highly recommended that you read it with him or her. It turns out that ADT can profoundly affect your relationships, so it is critical to address all parties concerned, not just the one receiving ADT.

This is not just a book that you read; it is a book that you *do*. It will serve as a reference and will complement whatever your medical team has taught you. It will allow you and your partner to better understand what is going on, and why, and it will help you to better deal with some of the side effects of ADT. It is a fantastic resource for patients and their families that is long overdue. As Sir Francis Bacon said in 1597, "knowledge is power." Get going on *doing* this book, and in the process take back the power that prostate cancer has been stealing from you. You'll be glad you did.

*Celestia (Tia) Higano, MD*
Professor, Medical Oncology Division
University of Washington, School of Medicine
Seattle, Washington

# Introduction

This book is designed to help prostate cancer patients and their loved ones learn about and deal with the side effects of androgen deprivation therapy (ADT), commonly referred to as hormone therapy. You may have already received some information from your physician, nurse, or pharma-

> Most patients tell us that they prefer to know about all possible side effects ahead of time, rather than be surprised by any side effects, even when there is only a small chance of experiencing them.

cist about the common side effects of ADT. This book will provide you with more information and prepare you for what you might experience while on ADT. Not all patients experience every side effect, and severity varies from patient to patient. We hope that by using this book you will be better able to adjust to ADT, cope with its impact on your life, and manage the side effects that you experience.

You may find that some strategies provided here seem like a good fit for you, while others do not. Use what works for you. It may be helpful to read the book at the start of treatment, or shortly before, and then again some months later. Material that may not have seemed relevant initially may become more so over time.

There is also information here for the loved ones of men on ADT. Some sections are appropriate for all loved ones; others are specifically for sexual partners.

Openly discussing the side effects can make it easier to adapt overall and may help you learn ways of managing the side effects so you have a better quality of life. It is important to discuss your concerns with your health care providers before you start ADT *and* during treatment.

- It is important to maintain open communication with your partner, family, and friends, as well as with your doctor and nurse.
- Keep your doctor updated about how you feel about the treatment and how you are dealing with the side effects.
- There is help available if you are struggling. Please don't wait until you are overwhelmed to ask for help.

## Before You Begin

We believe the value of this book is enhanced when patients and loved ones discuss ADT-related issues *together*. Questions at the end of each section are designed to help you think about how this information applies to you, and to facilitate communication with your loved ones. Some questions specifically address couples; others are appropriate for individuals, or for patients who are dating, or hope to date in the future. Even if you don't have a person you feel you can talk to about your concerns, we hope you will still think over these questions and answer them for your own benefit.

If you are currently in a relationship, we recommend that you and your partner work to maintain a strong, supportive bond with each other. This requires open and honest communication. If you are not in a relationship, you may consider asking a close friend or family member to discuss with you some of the topics that are raised in this book.

Here are some questions to consider before you begin. Try to answer all of them. There are no right or wrong answers. Taking time to reflect upon the questions, and writing down your answers, may be helpful. Use the space provided.

### Questions:
- What do I already know about ADT?
- What questions do I have about ADT?
- Which potential side effects are most concerning to me?
- What does it mean to me to be on ADT?
- Do I believe that being androgen-deprived will affect my sense of masculinity?
- How comfortable am I in talking about sex with my partner, a close friend, or with my physician?
- Who can I talk to about my concerns and about this book?

If you are in a relationship, some specific questions for couples include:

- How will our relationship change as a result of ADT?
- How might any changes affect my partner?
- Which changes concern me the most?
- What do we value most about our relationship?
- How comfortable are we talking to each other about sensitive issues, such as sex?
- How well do we communicate on a day-to-day basis?
- What areas of our communication could be improved?

**NOTES:**

_____

_____

_____

_____

_____

_____

_____

_____

_____

_____

_____

_____

_____

_____

_____

_____

_____

_____

### Will Reading This Book Make Me More or Less Anxious?

Some individuals are very laid back about gathering information on their illness and its management. Psychologists refer to such people as *blunters*. They generally take a relaxed approach to health care. They may seem less distressed, but they may miss out on critical information. Blunters may want only the essential information about ADT and find this book to be too detailed.

*Monitors*, on the other hand, are individuals who like to learn the details of a condition and all of the options available to them, including treatments and side effects—but they do tend to worry more. Monitors may want even more detail than what they will find here.

One style is not any better than the other. If you find that you and your partner have different styles, you can enlist each other's help. Knowing your tendencies and your partner's tendencies may help both of you deal with the challenges to come.

*If you are a blunter,* and the idea of reading the whole book is unappealing to you, here are some suggestions:

- Select certain parts to read by looking at the table of Contents or Index. Skim through the chapters, reading the topics that interest you the most.
- Read the questions at the end of each chapter.
- Ask someone to read the book and point out to you the sections that are most relevant.

*If you are a monitor,* you may appreciate how detailed this book is, but you may also find yourself getting anxious reading some parts. If you do, look for the reassuring messages throughout, and remember:

- Not all patients experience all side effects.

- There are many things that you can do to keep your body, mind, and relationship strong and healthy.
- There are steps you can take to manage the impact of ADT on you and your life.

### I Have Never Read a Manual Before—Why Start Now?

When we hand patients a copy of this book, they often say to us, "I have never read a manual before—why start now?" To help answer that question, here is a story drawn from our interactions with one particular patient. We hope his perspective encourages you to make the most of this book, instead of just skimming it.

*When my doctor said I should start hormone therapy, he told me I might have a few side effects, like hot flushes, gaining a few pounds, and I might lose interest in sex. He suggested I take vitamin D and calcium to keep my bones strong. That didn't sound too bad.*

*He also gave me this book and said it might help me deal with the side effects. I wasn't sure I needed to read it. I'd seen my wife deal with hot flushes, and we mostly just joked about it. I always ate healthy and walked the dog so I didn't think I had to worry about my weight. I'd been using Viagra since my surgery so we had already gotten used to not having sex like we used to. And I knew my marriage was solid. We've been together for 30 years— what is there that we couldn't handle? I'd dealt with lots of adversity in the past and over-come it, so I had every confidence that I would adapt this time too. Besides, I'd never read a manual before—I've always been able to figure things out on my own. Why start now?*

*I figured I would take things a day at a time, but I was surprised when the changes slowly crept up on me. I tried to joke about the hot flashes, but I was really embarrassed when I was in a business meeting and got all red in the face and broke out in a sweat. One day, when I got out of the shower, I really looked at myself in the mirror. Somehow, I had developed a beer belly. I'd always taken pride in being in good shape and here I'd put on 15 pounds, without even noticing.*

*That day, I looked at my body and saw that my penis had shrunk, and my testicles too! I was angry that no one told me that my genitals would shrink after beginning on hor-monal treatment. I started to feel really down about myself and my ability to satisfy my wife. Even though my mood started to tank, I told myself I needed to suck it up and not make a big deal of it.*

*I did my best to ignore these changes, but I started to notice that my wife seemed unhappy. I asked her what was wrong. She was very reluctant to say anything at first. I had to encourage her to say what was on her mind. She then started to point out how I had changed and how our relationship had changed. She said I had withdrawn from her both physically and emotionally. She told me she understood that I might not have the desire to have sex; what I didn't notice was that I had stopped regularly touching her. My kisses had become mechanical.*

*She feared we had become more like brother and sister than husband and wife. I had become grumpy and sometimes was short with her. I seemed tired and unenthusiastic about life. She went on to say that she was saddened by the changes and felt lonely, but was reluctant to bring this all up because she knew it wasn't my fault. She was patiently waiting, hoping that we would just adapt to these changes with time.*

*After my wife told me how she felt, I realized that I needed to do something. I didn't know what to do, so I started by calling my doctor's office. We got a referral to a counselor willing to talk with us. When my wife and I went to see the counselor, he asked if I'd read this book. I had to admit that I'd only glanced at it and hadn't really read it. In fact, I had forgotten all about it. I promised I would dig it out and read it before our next meeting.*

*I was surprised to learn in the book that there are things I could try to control the hot flashes. I learned about the importance of physical activity in keeping my weight under control and stopping the loss of muscle mass. I realized that there were things I could have been doing to help prevent myself from being in this situation.*

*Also, reading the material and doing the exercises with my wife was actually really helpful. It helped us to understand what was happening between us and what other couples on hormone therapy did to keep their relationship strong. I was surprised to learn how some couples even continue to enjoy sexual activity. Reading this book turned my life around. In hindsight, I think it could have helped to prevent a lot of suffering for both my wife and me.*

*I don't know why I was so reluctant to read it. I guess I had assumed that these things were not going to happen to me. I told one of my engineering friends that I wished I'd read the book back when I started on hormone therapy like my doctor had suggested. He asked, "Have you ever heard the expression RTFM?" I hadn't, so I went online and searched the term. Do you know what it stands for? If you don't know what it means, and won't be offended by strong language, you might want to do an online search too.*

*Perhaps this book should come with that recommendation, "RTFM," in bold letters. It may be crass, but it's advice best taken. My wife now makes a point of teasing me about it, and I have a good laugh when I make this recommendation to other men starting on this treatment.*

Although ADT injections are only given to the patient, the effects of ADT can produce physical and emotional changes in the patient that may indirectly affect his loved ones. The goal of this book is to help both patients and loved ones recognize and adapt to the side effects of ADT.

### Moving Forward: Questions for Discussion

Below are questions that should help you to reflect on the material in this section and how it may affect you. Try to answer each question.

- How do you react to illness in general—are you more of a monitor or a blunter?
- What have you already heard from either health care professionals or others about the side effects of ADT?
- Do you have specific questions that you would like to have answered about the form of ADT that you have been offered and the side effects of the treatment?
- Have you discussed with your physician how long you might need to be on ADT and whether you are a candidate for intermittent ADT?

**NOTES:**

_____

_____

_____

_____

_____

_____

_____

_____

_____

_____

_____

_____

_____

_____

_____

_____

_____

_____

_____

_____

_____

_____

_____

# I

# Androgen Deprivation Therapy

As a patient, you are about to begin treatment with drugs that reduce the amount of male hormones, called androgens, in your body. The main androgens are **testosterone\*** and **dihydrotestosterone** (DHT). This treatment, while commonly called hormone therapy, is more properly called androgen depri vation therapy or **ADT**.

## What is ADT?

ADT is effective in managing prostate cancer and treating the symptoms associated with prostate cancer. ADT works by reducing testosterone (produced in the testicles), the main **hormone** that stimulates the growth of prostate cancer cells. This can slow or even stop the spread of your prostate cancer and eliminate or significantly reduce the symptoms associated with the disease. Many men benefit, often for years, from ADT.

Testosterone affects many other tissues in the body in addition to the prostate gland, and a man on ADT will likely experience changes and side effects related to the lack of testosterone. Many patients and their loved ones readily accept the side effects of ADT in return for a life-prolonging treatment and recognize the trade-off between some quality of life for quantity of life. Other patients and their loved ones struggle to adjust to the side effects. We focus here on how you can maintain a good quality of life while on ADT.

ADT causes prostate cancer tumors to shrink, but may not kill them. It is thus understood as a treatment that is therapeutic, but usually not curative. Since it can significantly extend one's life, patients on ADT can view their

---

\*Technical terms are in bold in the text the first time they are used and are defined in the Glossary.

cancer as a chronic disease similar to high blood pressure or diabetes. For these conditions, medications are taken to manage, rather than to cure the illness. With good management of a chronic illness, even when primary treatment has failed, a patient can still expect to live a good, long life. A patient on ADT can realistically expect to live long enough to see further improvements in treatment. A cure may still be found. Starting on ADT does not mean that one will die of prostate cancer.

> Good management of chronic diseases, means changing one's lifestyle. The same can be said for living well on ADT.

## How Does ADT Work?

Androgen deprivation is commonly achieved by administering drugs (see the tables on the facing page) in the form of a simple injection. These injections contain a pellet which slowly releases synthetic hormones that block the chemical signal from the brain (specifically from a gland at the base of the brain called the **pituitary gland**) that normally tells the testicles to produce testosterone. The most common drugs used for ADT are called **LHRH agonists** or GnRH agonists (LHRH stands for luteinizing hormone-releasing hormone and GnRH stands for gonadotropin-releasing hormone, but they refer to the same thing). A different class of drugs called **GnRH antagonists** (or LHRH antagonists) can also shut down that signal to the testicles, with similar side effects.

With the injections, you may also be prescribed oral medications called **antiandrogens** (see the table in the following discussion). These drugs work differently, that is, by blocking the ability of testosterone (and other androgens) to attach to the cancer cells, thus preventing their growth.

Commonly, patients who are prescribed an LHRH agonist are advised to start taking an oral antiandrogen 2 to 3 weeks before getting their first LHRH agonist injection. For some patients it may be beneficial to stay on the antiandrogen long-term, but for others it may not be necessary. When an LHRH drug and an antiandrogen are taken together, they are often referred to as *combined androgen blockade* (CAB), *total androgen blockade* (TAB), or *maximum androgen blockade* (MAB). Some patients also refer to this combination as **ADT2**.

The table at the top of the facing page lists commonly prescribed LHRH drugs and their relevant information.

The second table on the facing page, "Antiandrogen Drugs Commonly Used to Treat Prostate Cancer," lists three commonly used antiandrogens that may be prescribed along with injectable medications to achieve CAB, or given to patients short-term for a few weeks before starting on an LHRH agonist.

There are other drugs being introduced into clinical practice and in research trials that also impact the hormonal environment in the body, including

**LHRH Drugs Commonly Used to Treat Prostate Cancer**

| Generic Name | Trade Name | How is the Drug Given?* | How Often is the Drug Given? |
|---|---|---|---|
| Leuprolide | Lupron® | Intramuscular injection | Every 1, 3, 4, or 6 months** |
| | Eligard® | Subcutaneous injection | Every 1, 3, 4, or 6 months** |
| Goserelin | Zoladex® | Subcutaneous injection | Every month or every 3 months** |
| Triptorelin | Trelstar® | Intramuscular injection | Every 1, 3, or 6 months** |
| Buserelin | Suprefact® | Subcutaneous injection | Every 3 months |
| | | Nasal spray | Daily |
| Degarelix | Firmagon® | Subcutaneous injection | Two initial injections and then monthly injections |

*Subcutaneous injections are given under the skin, usually in the abdomen. Intramuscular injections are usually injected into the muscle of the buttock.
**Frequency of injections depends on the dose.
Note: The dosage and location of injection may vary between drugs, but the long-term side effects are similar whether the drugs are agonists or antagonists (i.e., degarelix). After the injection is administered, you may feel tenderness and/or itchiness and a small lump under the skin at the injection site.

**Antiandrogen Drugs Commonly Used to Treat Prostate Cancer**

| Generic Name | Trade Name | How is the Drug Given? | How Often is the Drug Given? |
|---|---|---|---|
| Flutamide | Eulexin® | Pill | Three times daily |
| Bicalutamide | Casodex® | Pill | Daily |
| Nilutamide | Nilandron® (United States) | Pill | Daily |
| | Anandron® (Canada) | Pill | Daily |

enzalutamide (Xtandi®) and abiraterone (Zytiga®). These will have an increasing role to play in the management of prostate cancer in the years to come. Enzalutamide is a new antiandrogen. Abiraterone is a drug that blocks testosterone production, not only from the testicles but also from the adrenal glands. Drugs like abiraterone are so effective in reducing testosterone that they have been referred to in the recent medical literature as causing "androgen annihilation" rather than androgen deprivation. There are many promising studies looking at early use of these two compounds as alternatives to LHRH drugs.

Although not commonly used in North America as a first-line hormone therapy, female hormones called **estrogens** can also be used to suppress testosterone. These can be either natural (e.g., **estradiol**) or synthetic (e.g., diethylstilbestrol [DES]) compounds. At high concentrations, like the LHRH drugs, they can reduce the hormonal signals from the brain to the testicles to produce testosterone. The oral forms of these drugs have been associated with an elevated risk of blood clot formation and are rarely used in North America and Europe. However, if taken nonorally, such as through the skin (e.g., by patch or gel), the risk is much lower. Research is underway to see if they are as effective in cancer control and with fewer bothersome side effects than the LHRH drugs. At low doses, estrogenic compounds can help reduce some of the side effects of the LHRH drugs.

### What Medications Are You Taking for ADT?

The chart below can help you to track the ADT drugs that have been prescribed for you. An additional copy is available in the Appendix on page 120.

| Medication | Dose | How Often? |
|---|---|---|
|  |  |  |
|  |  |  |
|  |  |  |
|  |  |  |
|  |  |  |

### Testosterone and Dihydrotestosterone

Some of the testosterone in a man's body is converted to another androgen called dihydrotestosterone (DHT). DHT also binds to receptors on prostate cells like testosterone and is a more potent stimulus for the growth of prostate cancer cells.

Medications that block the conversion of testosterone to DHT, such as finasteride (Proscar®) and dutasteride (Avodart®), are often prescribed to manage symptoms related to benign enlargement of the prostate (called *benign prostatic hypertrophy*, or BPH). Both are oral medications. The benefits of these medications in managing prostate cancer are uncertain. Some patients may be prescribed these drugs to help with urinary complaints. Some clinicians and patients refer to using this drug together with LHRH agonists and anti-androgens as "triple blockade," or **ADT3**. There is no clinical evidence that

ADT3 is significantly more effective at controlling prostate cancer than the LHRH drugs used alone or with an antiandrogen.

## How Long Will I Be on ADT?

The duration of ADT recommended to you will depend upon your situation. *Life-long ADT* is prescribed in either of these two circumstances:

1. PSA continues to rise after completion of primary treatments, such as **prostatectomy, brachytherapy,** or **radiotherapy.**
2. Your cancer is known to have spread beyond the prostate.

Some patients are on ADT for a while, and then stop and take a "drug holiday." Cycling on and off the drug is known as *intermittent hormonal therapy.* Whether intermittent therapy is the best program for you will depend upon how well your cancer is controlled and how your **prostate-specific antigen (PSA)** level behaves over time. The case for "going intermittent" is that for many patients it can limit the side effects of treatment, while still maintaining good overall long-term cancer control.

*Short-term ADT* is often recommended, from six months up to three years, for patients with cancer confined to the prostate gland who go for some form of radiotherapy as a primary treatment. In this situation, ADT is often given for a few months prior to the start of the radiation therapy and continued throughout the radiotherapy treatment period, as well as for several months afterward. These patients may be recommended to stay on the drugs longer if their cancer appears to be a bit more aggressive. However, newer studies suggest that ADT, when given to enhance radiotherapy, can be effective for many patients when administered for a shorter period of time, ranging from 6 to 18 months.

## What Is the PSA Test?

PSA is a protein produced by cells of the prostate gland. The **PSA test** measures the level of PSA in a man's blood. For this test, a blood sample is sent to a laboratory for analysis. PSA is present in small quantities in the blood of men with healthy prostates, but is often elevated in the presence of prostate cancer or other prostate disorders.

### How is the PSA Test Used for Men Who Have Been Treated for Prostate Cancer?

An increase in PSA in a patient who has had treatment for prostate cancer *may* be a sign of a recurrence of the disease. A single elevated PSA in a patient who has a history of prostate cancer is not a guarantee of recurrent cancer, and it is often necessary to repeat PSA testing over time to identify trends before confirming recurrence of the disease. Such recurrence is called a *biochemical relapse* if (a) the PSA rises over time, and if (b) examination and diagnostic imaging (e.g., computed tomography [CT] or bone scans) do not identify tumor deposits related to prostate cancer. If the examination or diagnostic imaging shows that there has been a spread of the cancer, it is called *metastatic disease*.

### How is the PSA Test Used When You Are on ADT?

A PSA that remains low indicates that your cancer is being controlled. If you are on intermittent therapy, ADT is stopped when the PSA drops to a very low level. If the PSA level rises above a specific threshold, ADT is started again. How high the PSA is allowed to rise before stopping or starting back on ADT is a matter to discuss with your physician.

### How Good Is the PSA Test?

The PSA level is a good indicator of the effectiveness of treatment. Generally speaking, your PSA should be very low while on ADT, but this can vary. The PSA level itself does not predict whether or not a man will have symptoms or how long the man will live. Many men have very high PSA values and feel just fine. Other men have low values yet have symptoms of the disease. PSA levels are *not* a definitive measure of how serious one's prostate cancer is and are only part of the information that your doctor uses to determine how you are doing in relation to your prostate cancer.

PSA levels normally fluctuate in all men. Many men dealing with prostate cancer are understandably concerned about even very small changes in their PSA. For men whose cancer has recurred or spread outside the prostate gland, the actual PSA level is typically not as important as how quickly it rises. However, not every rise in PSA means that the cancer is growing and requires treatment right away. To help avoid unnecessary anxiety, be sure you understand what level of change in your PSA is considered a cause for concern. You can determine this by speaking with your doctor.

## How Long Will ADT Control My Cancer?

Patients may be treated with ADT for many years, for as long as it is beneficial in managing their cancer. Many men have been on ADT for more than a decade. ADT works for varying periods of time in different patients. Be sure to discuss with your doctor your questions about the duration of ADT and the potential for intermittent treatment strategies. Intermittent therapy requires regular monitoring of your PSA and overall health to ensure that drug treatments are reinitiated in a timely fashion if necessary. Intermittent therapy appears to maintain the benefits of hormonal treatment for prostate cancer, and is associated with a better quality of life during the "off" treatment periods.

However, over time ADT will likely become less effective at reducing PSA levels. When that happens, other treatments (e.g., second-line hormonal therapies) can be considered. Long-term administration of ADT is increasingly offered to patients in the intermittent manner. This cyclic use of the LHRH drugs is thought to prolong the length of time that the ADT remains effective in controlling the cancer.

Hearing that your primary treatment did not get rid of all the cancer or that your cancer has spread can be distressing for both you and your loved ones. At this point, we know that the previous, potentially curative treatment has failed. Some distress is understandable in this situation. These feelings should be balanced against the reality that ADT can help control your cancer for a long time, and patients now on intermittent ADT may go through a half dozen or more "off" cycles, which can sometimes span a decade or longer.

For patients on intermittent ADT, getting PSA tests and waiting for the results are often stressful times. Feeling nervous or anxious is realistic in response to this difficult situation. However, if you find that you are significantly distressed at any time while being treated with ADT—whether on an "on" or "off" cycle—you should consider asking your medical team for help in dealing with the stress. Please share your concerns with your physician or seek professional counseling.

A chart for tracking your PSA scores throughout your treatment is provided below and an additional copy is located in the Appendix on page 121.

**PSA Chart:** Write down the results from your PSA tests to keep track of any changes.

| Date | PSA Level | Date | PSA Level | Date | PSA Level |
|------|-----------|------|-----------|------|-----------|
|      |           |      |           |      |           |
|      |           |      |           |      |           |
|      |           |      |           |      |           |
|      |           |      |           |      |           |
|      |           |      |           |      |           |

## Moving Forward: Questions for Discussion

- Are there questions that I have about ADT for my health care team?
- Am I on continuous or intermittent ADT?
- Do I know my PSA?
- Does getting my PSA checked and waiting for results make me nervous or anxious?

## NOTES:

_____

_____

_____

_____

_____

_____

_____

_____

_____

_____

_____

_____

_____

_____

_____

# 2

# Physical Side Effects

ADT eliminates most of the testosterone in a man's body. This can lead to many physical side effects. This chapter covers the various side effects that you may experience and offers suggestions for dealing with them. Some of these effects are similar to those experienced by women when they reach menopause. This comparison may help loved ones understand what men on ADT experience.

## Hot Flashes

*Hot flashes* (also called *hot flushes*) are often listed by patients as one of the most bothersome side effects of ADT. As many as 80% of ADT patients may experience hot flashes. Hot flashes can occur within three weeks of starting ADT, and may or may not decrease in frequency over the duration of ADT. Many men report that they get used to hot flashes and are better able to cope with them over time.

Hot flashes feel like waves of heat in the face, head, and upper body. Hot flashes involve the perception of heat and are not associated with any substantial increase in body temperature. A hot flash may last for less than three minutes, and you may feel uncomfortably warm. A severe hot flash can make you feel very hot and sweaty, and you may feel as if you need to change your clothes or bedding.

Hot flashes are often associated with sweating. When the sweating occurs at night, this is called a *night sweat*. Night sweats can interfere with the *quality* of sleep and lead to daytime fatigue, even if you don't remember having them. Night sweats may not only disrupt your sleep, but may also disrupt the sleep of your partner. Treatments for hot flashes may thus help improve sleep quality and reduce daytime fatigue for both of you. Even if you aren't sure whether hot flashes are disrupting your sleep, you may want to explore with your physician whether a treatment for hot flashes might help with any fatigue you are experiencing.

A hot flash will pass. When you experience one, it can help to use a cold compress, or fan yourself (paper and battery-operated hand-held fans are easy to use and portable). If hot flashes occur often, wear loose clothing in layers that can be quickly put on or taken off. Hot flashes may also improve if you:

- Quit smoking.
- Reduce the amount of spicy food you eat.
- Keep your room at a cooler temperature and use a fan.
- Use light bedding and/or a towel on your sheets.
- Wear breathable (cotton or merino wool) clothing.
- Take warm, rather than hot, baths and showers.

There is some evidence that acupuncture may help reduce the frequency and duration of hot flashes.

Ingesting soy may also help reduce hot flashes. Compounds derived from plants (e.g., black cohosh, soybean products), are often suggested as "natural" treatments for hot flashes. None, however, have been shown to be effective in properly designed clinical trials. For more information, see Chapter 4 on healthy eating.

The research demonstrating effectiveness of these treatments is often drawn from the experiences of women with hot flashes at menopause. Less research has been undertaken with men, and some treatments effective for women may be less effective for men on ADT.

We have heard from some patients that they are actually pleased to experience hot flashes, as it confirms for them that the androgen deprivation treatment is really working. However, although it is true that hot flashes are an indication of androgen suppression, it would be a mistake to think that there is a relationship between how many hot flashes one experiences and how effective androgen deprivation is in controlling one's cancer. The fact is that there is no benefit in enduring hot flashes that disrupt one's life day and night.

If hot flashes or night sweats are distressing to you and/or interfere with your sleep, speak to your doctor about medications that can help. Here are some options to consider (also see the table on p. 12).

### Medications

- **Estradiol**, the most common natural estrogen, can be applied in low doses to the skin. Many women use this as part of *hormone replacement therapy* to reduce hot flashes during menopause. Estradiol works the same way for men on ADT. Estradiol is available by prescription only. The two forms are:

- Adhesive patches that stick to your skin, applied on your buttocks or belly. The patches last up to a week so you don't need to bother with them for days at a time, but they may irritate the skin or become visible by picking up dye from your clothing.
- A gel that you can spread on your arms, legs, or abdomen that is clear and quick-drying, so it is not visible, but must be applied daily.

*Note:* This treatment should be used with caution if there is a family history of breast cancer that is estrogen-sensitive. Men should be aware that high dose estradiol may cause enlargement of their breasts and nipple sensitivity. Also, based on what is known about estrogens taken orally at a high dose, there remains a potential risk of blood clots. Although that has not been reported in prostate cancer patients applying estradiol to their skin, it really has not been investigated extensively in men on ADT.

- Venlafaxine (Effexor®), a commonly used antidepressant, can help control hot flashes when prescribed in small doses. Venlafaxine is one drug in a class of drugs called *serotonin norepinephrine reuptake inhibitors* (SNRIs). Other drugs in this class can also be helpful.
- Gabapentin (Neurontin®) is a drug commonly used to treat epilepsy and certain types of chronic pain. It has been shown to be moderately effective in treating hot flashes in men on ADT. However, it has not been shown to be better than the agents mentioned above.

There are other drugs that have been shown to help reduce hot flashes in women but have not been well studied in prostate cancer patients on ADT. A couple of these drugs, medroxyprogesterone (Provera®) and megestrol (Megace®), are derived from another natural female hormone, progesterone. Progesterone-derived medications are best known for being used in birth control pills and to treat certain female cancers.

- Medroxyprogesterone is primarily a long-acting birth control agent for women (given as an injected drug known as Depo-Provera®), but has also been used at high doses to lower the sex drive in sex offenders. The fact that it has to be injected makes it less convenient than a pill or a drug applied to the skin. While progesterone-derived agents can reduce hot flashes, they have other side effects that can add to, rather than reduce, the overall side effects of the LHRH drugs.
- There are case reports that megestrol has stimulated cancer and, therefore, if it is used to treat hot flashes, the cancer needs to be followed closely for signs of progression. Although it can suppress hot flashes, it also may cause weight gain.

Listed below are prescription drugs used to treat hot flashes.

**Some Medications for ADT-Induced Hot Flashes**

| Generic Name | Trade Name | How Is the Drug Given? | How Often Is the Drug Given? |
|---|---|---|---|
| Estradiol | EstroGel® | Gel | Rubbed on the arm once a day |
| | Alora® | Patch | Applied weekly or twice weekly on the lower abdomen or buttocks |
| | Climara® Dermestril® Elleste Solo® Esclim® Menostar® Vivelle-Dot® | | |
| Venlafaxine | Effexor | Pill | Depends on the dose and formulation |
| Gabapentin | Neurontin | Pill | Depends on the dose and formulation |
| Medroxyprogesterone | Provera | Intramuscular injection into the thigh, abdomen, or arm | One injection every 3 months |
| Megestrol | Megace | Pill | Depends on the dose and formulation |

## Counseling

Counseling approaches such as *cognitive behavioral therapy*, can also help you better adjust to the distress (e.g., panic or anger) of experiencing a hot flash and to deal with negative opinions about what it means to experience a hot flash. The breathing exercise below is an example of a behavioral technique that has been shown to help coping with hot flashes. The hot flash diary on page 14 is an example of a cognitive technique for coping with distressing thoughts about hot flashes.

## Activity: Abdominal Breathing

Another technique used to reduce hot flashes is called *abdominal breathing*, or *paced respiration*, which can be used both to reduce the frequency of hot flashes and as a relaxation technique. This type of breathing is most effective after you have practiced it regularly:

- Sit comfortably and place one hand on your belly and one on your chest.
- When you are breathing deeply and slowly, you will find that your belly moves up and down more than if you were taking shallow breaths.
- When you are ready, take a deep breath in through your nose. Make this inhalation last for a count of four, and then pause. Breathe out through your nose, exhaling out all the breath while slowly counting to four, and then pause. Inhale. Exhale. Inhale. Exhale. Try doing this for a few minutes.
- Be sure to focus on your breath. If you notice thoughts coming and going, simply acknowledge them and bring your attention back to your breath. If you get overwhelmed, tired, or dizzy at first, take a break for about 30 seconds and continue when you are ready. It helps to concentrate on slowly filling and emptying your lungs as fully as is possible.

With continued practice (daily, for 5 minutes at a time), you can get better at this activity and it can be an effective, simple, way to cope with a hot flash. This is also an effective strategy for coping with anxiety and stress, discussed further in Chapter 5.

### Activity: Hot Flash Diary

You may find a hot flash diary to be helpful for tracking the frequency of your hot flashes, how bothersome they are to you, and how you will cope with them. Sometimes the thoughts that come with hot flashes can be as distressing as the hot flash itself. For example, if you think, "Oh no, I can't cope with this hot flash," this mere thought can perpetuate distress. It may be helpful to challenge this thought or remind yourself of a coping statement. Examples of these include:

"There are things I can do to cope with this discomfort, such as deep breathing."
"The people I am with right now know what I am going through and are not going to judge me for having a hot flash."
"Getting worked up about the hot flash won't do anything to help it."
"I can ask my doctor about medications to help with hot flashes."

Coping statements give a rational perspective on the situation and are helpful in handling momentary distress. They help keep distressing thoughts in check and prevent a person from becoming overwhelmed by them. Keeping a record of your hot flashes can help increase objectivity and thus decrease distress. You can find the hot flash diary on the next page, as well as in the Appendix on page 122.

**Hot Flash Diary**

| Day | Intensity (0–10) | Duration | Distressing Thought/ Appraisal | Coping Statement |
|---|---|---|---|---|
| Sunday | | | | |
| Monday | | | | |
| Tuesday | | | | |
| Wednesday | | | | |
| Thursday | | | | |
| Friday | | | | |
| Saturday | | | | |

## Weaker Bones

ADT can affect your bones. Slight weakening of bones is called *osteopenia*; more extensive weakening is called **osteoporosis**. With weaker bones, the risk of breaking a bone is increased. If there is a history of osteoporosis or hip fractures in your family, you may be at even higher risk while on ADT. Here are some things you can do before and while you are on ADT to prevent osteoporosis and bone fractures:

● Get a baseline bone density exam, before or very shortly after starting ADT, and discuss with your doctor what actions you can take to reduce your risk of osteoporosis. This test is simple, noninvasive, and can be repeated over time to assess the impact of ADT on your bone health.

● See Chapter 3 on exercise for activities that will help strengthen bones and improve muscle strength and balance.

● Stop smoking and limit alcohol and caffeine consumption.

● Maintain a healthy weight.

- Talk to your doctor about taking calcium and vitamin D supplementation. You should aim for 600 to 800 **IU** (International Units) of vitamin D a day (described in more detail in Chapter 4).

- Bisphosphonates are a class of drugs commonly used to treat osteoporosis and may be used to counteract the effects of ADT on your bones. These agents may also be helpful in managing prostate cancer that has spread to your bones. Orally and intravenously administered forms of these drugs can be used. Like any medication, there are potential side effects and risks associated with the use of bisphosphonates that you should be aware of and discuss with your doctor before starting on treatment.

- If you are starting on drug treatments to protect your bones, it is important to make your dentist aware and to have a dental assessment because of a rare, yet potentially serious side effect called *osteonecrosis of the jaw* (ONJ). Your dentist can take precautions to reduce the risk of ONJ.

- Long-term use (e.g., five years or more) of bisphosphonates for postmenopausal women has been shown to occasionally lead to a rare form of hip or thigh fracture. If you are taking a bisphosphonate for a long time and experience hip pain, be sure to bring that to the attention of your physician.

- Using transdermal estradiol to reduce hot flashes may also help keep your bones strong.

- Denosumab (Xgeva®) is a drug that can be used to help manage bone health in patients with osteoporosis and in patients whose cancer is affecting their bones. Denosumab is given once every six months to men with osteoporosis. However, for patients whose cancer has spread (i.e., is metastatic) it may be given more often, such as once a month, for as long as it is needed. It can, however, interfere with immune function, slightly increasing the risk of respiratory or bladder infections and, like the bisphosphonates, it carries a small risk of ONJ.

### Weight Gain and Muscle Loss

Weight gain is a common complaint of many men who are treated with ADT. An increase in body fat mass up to 10% is not uncommon, with much of the new weight added around the abdomen and hips. If you are presently at a normal or low weight, weight gain of this amount may not be serious. However, if you are already overweight, relatively inactive, or at risk of developing diabetes,

> Well-structured exercise programs are prescribed treatments for many medical conditions. Unless you have been told by your doctor not to exercise, we encourage you to view an exercise program as a significant part of your treatment regimen while on ADT. We recognize that starting a program now may not be easy, but its benefits are many!

then weight gain may be problematic. Increases in weight while on ADT can lead to medical complications, such as diabetes and cardiac problems (called **metabolic syndrome**).

Weight gain related to ADT is typically associated with a loss of 3% to 4% of muscle mass. As a combination, it makes moving more difficult, and being inactive just makes the problem worse. If you are not already exercising consistently, try increasing your activity level gradually. If you find yourself gaining a lot of weight, one of the best things you can do is maintain a regular exercise schedule. See Chapter 3 on exercise for more information. Suggestions for implementing your exercise routine include:

- Joining a structured program at a gym or community center.
- Purchasing equipment to use at home, such as small free weights and stretchable bands.

> It is important that you do not wait until you notice changes in weight and muscle mass before you begin an exercise program. **Start now!** You may find it more enjoyable to pursue an exercise program with your partner, a friend, or a loved one.

## Diabetes

ADT not only increases the risk of adult onset (type 2) diabetes, but has also recently been found to make the control of diabetes with medications alone more difficult. Thus, prostate cancer patients who are diabetic and starting on ADT need to be particularly concerned about their lifestyle (i.e., diet and exercise) if they are going to keep the diabetes under control and avoid the more serious complications of that disease.

Active research is underway to find out whether patients on ADT do better if given medicine to treat diabetes preemptively. Although not all the results are in yet, a patient on ADT who is already diabetic or at particularly high risk of developing that disease, may want to discuss with his physician the pros and cons of taking a drug for diabetes while on ADT. One drug that has been used to treat diabetes is metformin (sold as Glucophage®, Fortamet®, Glumetza®, or Riomet®) and it may be helpful to patients on ADT as well. *However*, taking such a drug is *not* a replacement for exercising. As noted above, the effectiveness of such drugs is already known to be better for patients who are actively exercising.

## Metabolic Syndrome and Cardiovascular Risk

ADT has been shown to cause metabolic abnormalities. **Metabolic syndrome** involves three of the following five symptoms: increased blood sugar (higher than 110 mg/dL), increased triglycerides (150 mg/dL or higher), low high-density lipoproteins (less than 40 mg/dL), increased waist circumference of 40 inches (102 cm), and/or increased blood pressure (130/85 mmHg or higher).

Men on ADT often experience an increase in blood sugar, triglycerides, and waist circumference, and as such, ADT could increase cardiovascular disease risk.

## Anemia and Fatigue

From a third to a half of men on ADT experience some level of daytime fatigue. This effect seems to be felt more by younger men, since they experience a greater drop in testosterone. There may be several causes for this. ADT can, for example, cause mild anemia (low red blood cell count). You may be suffering from night sweats (hot flashes) that are disrupting your sleep. There is also mental fatigue associated with ADT (see Chapter 5). As a result, you may feel less motivated to exercise or participate in physical activities. You may also get out of breath more quickly when you are physically active. You may not feel like exercising because you are too tired, *but the single best way to combat fatigue from ADT is through exercise.*

*Note:* ADT-associated anemia is *not* due to an iron deficiency. Taking an iron supplement is *not* recommended unless you are iron-deficient.

Avoiding exercise is a vicious circle: you will lose muscle mass and gain weight, which makes you feel more tired and even less enthusiastic about exercising. You may feel that exercising isn't helping; you may still gain weight and lose muscle mass despite exercising. That doesn't mean that exercise is not preventing things from being much worse. Read Chapter 3 on exercise and talk with your physician to find an exercise program that is best for you.

> Regular exercise reduces fatigue, keeps muscles strong, and limits weight gain. It promotes an all-around better mood during the day and helps improve sleep quality.

## Breast Growth

Approximately 15% of patients taking LHRH agonists experience some level of breast enlargement and increased breast sensitivity. Such breast growth in men is called **gynecomastia**. The amount of breast growth is usually slight, but the nipples and surrounding skin may become more sensitive to touch. Gynecomastia is more common in patients taking antiandrogen medications that may be prescribed to enhance ADT effectiveness. It is also common in patients who may use estradiol to reduce hot flashes. Some patients find that they are uncomfortable with the changes in appearance or nipple sensitivity that accompany gynecomastia. There is no way to predict who will experience these symptoms, but if you are overweight, your chances may be greater.

For most men, breasts are a major signifier of feminization, so any enlargement of their breasts is seen as loss of masculinity, identity, and status. Other men are not bothered by the changes. Some men even find the fact that they have gynecomastia amusing. If you stop ADT, breast sensitivity may stop, but the breast tissue itself will not disappear. If you are distressed by gynecomastia, you can:

- Wear a T-shirt at the gym or beach, or a wetsuit vest in the water.
- Exercise at home by investing in personal fitness equipment.
- Invest in garments that compress and flatten the chest, such as compression shirts.

> One man on ADT was able to joke about his breast development, teasing his wife that his breasts were younger and better looking than hers.

It is important that you and your intimate partner discuss what gynecomastia would mean to each of you. If you think that breast development will be very distressing to you, or that you cannot tolerate it at all, discuss preventative options with your doctor as soon as possible. Unfortunately, such procedures may not be covered by your health insurance.

An antiestrogen drug used to treat breast cancer, called tamoxifen (sold as Nolvadex®, Istubal®, or Valodex®), has been suggested as a way to prevent gynecomastia in men on ADT. However, research to date has not considered the potentially beneficial effects of estrogens in men on ADT. Until more is known about the side effects of tamoxifen in androgen-deprived men, this treatment is not recommended.

Some of the more established options to prevent or reduce gynecomastia include:

- *Irradiation of the breasts*: In order to be most effective, this treatment is offered to the patient *before* gynecomastia develops. The radiation decreases potential breast growth, and, to some extent, may help to reduce breast sensitivity and discomfort.
- *Breast reduction surgery*: If breast growth is very distressing, breast reduction surgery is an option, and in some cases may be covered by health insurance. There are various ways that this surgery can be performed. When it is performed for men with strictly cosmetic reasons, it can usually be done as a nipple-sparing (subcutaneous) mastectomy or with liposuction.

## Genital Shrinkage

With ADT, some shrinkage of the penis and testicles is common. The shrinkage of the testicles is directly related to the shutdown of their functions of producing testosterone and sperm. If you are on ADT short-term (less than three years), the size of your testicles can recover partially, or even fully, when your testosterone levels recover. Since the testicles are inside the scrotum and not externally visible, their shrinkage is usually less of an issue for men on ADT compared to the loss of penis length and girth.

If you have residual **erectile dysfunction (ED)** from an earlier treatment for prostate cancer (e.g., surgery or radiation), you may have already experienced some shrinkage of your penis. Along with a decrease in sex drive, men on ADT often lose the ability to have a strong and prolonged erection, including spontaneous erections, such as nocturnal erections. Just as the muscles in an arm will shrink if the arm is not flexed, the penis will shrink if erections become rare or disappear completely. Most often these changes occur slowly and may not be noticeable for many months.

> Whether or not you and your partner intend to engage in penetrative sex, it is important that you think about the impact that genital shrinkage will have on your self-image. Men vary greatly in how much their penis size means to their self-image.

Penile shrinkage combined with weight gain may make it more difficult to see the penis and accurately aim while urinating. If that becomes a problem, the solution is to urinate sitting down.

Genital shrinkage does not often get discussed with patients, but it is common among men who are on ADT long-term. Men's responses to genital shrinkage vary greatly. To some it is of no concern; while for others it is a major concern. Sexual partners respond differently as well. Even though many partners indicate that penis size does not matter to them, they should appreciate that it can be an emotionally charged issue for some men.

If you do not envision participating in penetrative sex in the future, penis size and function may not be an issue for you. Still, you may be concerned about how your penis looks or feels to you, even if function is not an issue. For some men, such an alteration can really affect their self-esteem. If distress about this change prevents you from living well and especially from going to the gym or the swimming pool, schedule your exercise program so you can shower and dress in private.

If penis size is important to you, and if your hormone treatment is short-term, and if you envision resuming intercourse when you are off of ADT, you may want to read about options to maintain penis size and/or function in the absence of erections. Several management strategies are available, including ways to create erections regularly (such as the use of a vacuum erection device [VED] or penile injection) that can help keep the penile tissues from shrinking. Certain erectile dysfunction treatments can produce erections even in the absence of strong sexual desire. It should be acknowledged, though, that in the absence of a strong libido, artificially induced erections may feel mechanical and unnatural to a patient.

You and your sexual partner may wish to research erectile dysfunction treatments. We encourage you to read the whole chapter on intimacy and sexuality, starting on page 83. It is important to note that not all men who try these strategies find them helpful or effective.

## Loss of Body Hair

Men on ADT typically lose the hair on their chest, back, arms, and legs. Hair in the armpits and facial hair may be reduced in density, but hair on the top of the head and pubic hair remain. There are no physical health implications to losing body hair, and there is no easy way to stop it. Be aware that many men nowadays spend a lot of effort shaving and waxing to remove body hair, and men vary enormously on how hairy their bodies are to begin with. Thus, reduced body hair may even go unnoticed by those other than yourself or intimate partners.

## Other Possible Side Effects

The pharmaceutical literature on LHRH/GnRH agonists lists a few other physical side effects that infrequently occur, that is, in fewer than 10% of people, which is about the same for people who are not on ADT. These include joint or muscle pain and periodontal disease (the latter is a rare side effect, but nonetheless patients on ADT should take good care of their teeth and gums).

One recent study suggests that patients on ADT have a slightly increased risk of kidney disease. There are standard blood markers that indicate one's risk. As such, you may want to request that indicators of kidney function be included when you get your regular prostate-specific antigen (PSA) blood tests.

On an interesting note, one side effect that scientists are just now investigating is a decrease in body odor. This is simply mentioned here for thoroughness.

## Activity: Pros/Cons Table

Managing the side effects of ADT often requires making substantial changes to one's lifestyle. Sometimes, even though you *want* to make a lifestyle change, you may need to persuade yourself that the change is in fact worthwhile. A Pros/Cons table is a great way to convince yourself of the importance of making a change. You can redo it anytime you feel as if your life and priorities have shifted. Here's an example of a table:

| | PROS | CONS |
|---|---|---|
| **MAKING THE CHANGE:**<br>Walking daily | • Becoming fit<br>• Feeling better about myself<br>• Being outdoors<br>• Treats fatigue<br>• Helps treat muscle mass loss | • Requires effort<br>• Takes up time<br>• Tiring |
| **STAYING THE SAME:**<br>Stay at the same level of physical activity | • Easier to just enjoy myself and relax/sit on my couch<br>• Not tiring<br>• More time for other things | • I will probably gain weight<br>• I'm just so tired |

Now, try it out for yourself. An additional copy is in the Appendix on page 123.

| | PROS | CONS |
|---|---|---|
| **MAKING THE CHANGE:** | | |
| | | |
| **STAYING THE SAME:** | | |

## Activity: Action Plan

Throughout this book, there are suggestions for change that will help you and your partner maintain a high quality of life while on ADT. Are you thinking about making a lifestyle change? Eating better? Exercising more? Spending more time communicating with your partner? An *Action Plan* is a structured way to help you be clear about your goals, and increase the likelihood that you will follow through on your plans. It helps to be specific about when and where you plan to do the particular activity. You may wish to start small with something very manageable (e.g., going to the gym twice a week) before you take on larger-scale goals (e.g., going to the gym every-day). Discussing your Action Plan with a close friend or family member may help to keep you on track with your goals. Here is an example of a completed Action Plan:

**Action Plan Example: Practice Abdominal Breathing to Help with Hot Flashes**

**What I plan to do**:  try abdominal breathing for hot flashes

**When I plan to do it**:  twice a day before lunch and dinner

**Who I might do it with**:  by myself

**Why my plan is important**:  to help myself cope with discomfort

**Where I plan to do it**:  at my desk before lunch and/or in my living room before dinner

**What might get in the way?**  forgetting

**How I will address what might get in the way**:  I will put it on my schedule

Here is a blank copy that you can fill out. It helps to be as specific as possible when you are making your Action Plan. An additional copy is available in the Appendix on page 124.

**Action plan:** _____

What I plan to do: _____

_____

When I plan to do it: _____

_____

Who I might do it with: _____

_____

Why my plan is important: _____

_____

Where I plan to do it: _____

_____

What might get in the way? _____

_____

How I will address what might get in the way: _____

_____

## Activity: Goal Setting and Confidence • • • • • • • • • • • • • •

In order to support your goal, it can be helpful to ask yourself how confident you are that you can be successful in making this change. First, write down your goal (this might be what you have written in your Action Plan):

**GOAL #1** _____

i) Rate how confident you feel that you will achieve your goal:

   1      2      3      4      5      6      7      8      9      10

Not confident                           Very confident

ii) Rate how motivated you are to accomplish your goal:

   1      2      3      4      5      6      7      8      9      10

Not motivated                        Very motivated

iii) Rate how likely you are to actually carry out your goal:

   1      2      3      4      5      6      7      8      9      10

Not likely                            Very likely

If any of your answers *are less than 5*:

- Some ways to enhance motivation: (a) Consider enlisting the help of a friend to hold you accountable, (b) Set up a reward system, so that when you have achieved the goal, you can reward yourself, (c) Review a list of the possible benefits that may come from this change in behavior.
- Consider revising your goal—is it too ambitious? Can you start with a more modest goal and work your way up to a more significant lifestyle change?
- Remind yourself—What are the reasons why you are motivated to make this change?
- Consider completing the previous Pros/Cons table to help you identify your motivations (pros) for making this change, but also some of the barriers (cons) that might be getting in the way of making the change.

## Activity: Side Effects Self-Assessment • • • • • • • • • • • • • • • •

It is hard to adapt to changes one doesn't see or recognize. Thus, it's important to keep track of your side effects. Most of the side effects listed below were discussed in the current chapter, though a few are detailed more in Chapters 5 through 7. Awareness of change is always an aid in adapting to change. Use the questionnaire on the following page to help you recognize the impact of ADT on your life. Many of these side effects will take some time to develop; therefore, you may find it helpful to complete this brief assessment *after* you have been on ADT for three months. Fill it out and show it to your health care provider at your next appointment so that any concerns you have can be addressed. You may find it helpful to fill out the questionnaire before each of your medical appointments.

For descriptions and management strategies of the side effects listed below, see the appropriate chapter. You can find an additional copy of the side effect assessment in the Appendix on pages 126 to 127.

1. **During the past month**, how often have you experienced hot flashes? (*Please circle one number*).
   (1) More than once a day
   (2) About once a day
   (3) More than once a week
   (4) About once a week
   (5) Rarely or never

2. **During the past month**, how often have you had breast tenderness/sensitivity? (*Please circle one number*).
   (1) More than once a day
   (2) About once a day
   (3) More than once a week
   (4) About once a week
   (5) Rarely or never

3. **During the past month**, have you noticed any breast enlargement? (*Please circle one number*).
   (1) None
   (2) Minimal
   (3) Substantial
   (4) Moderate

4. **During the past month**, how much has your weight changed, if at all? (*Please circle one number*).
   (1) Gained 10 pounds/ 4.5 kilograms or more
   (2) Gained less than 10 pounds/ 4.5 kilograms
   (3) No change in weight
   (4) Lost less than 10 pounds/ 4.5 kilograms
   (5) Lost 10 pounds /4.5 kilograms or more

5. **During the past month**, have you experienced a change in the amount of hair on your arms, legs, and torso? (*Please circle one number*).
   (1) Loss of body hair on arms, legs and/or torso
   (2) No loss of body hair

6. **During the past month**, how concerned have you been about changes in how your penis and scrotum look? (*Please circle one number*).
   (1) Not concerned
   (2) A little concerned
   (3) Moderately concerned
   (4) Highly concerned

7. **During the past month**, how has your level of sexual desire been? (*Please circle one number*).
   (1) Very low to none
   (2) Low
   (3) Moderate
   (4) High
   (5) Very high

8. **During the past month**, how has your ability to have an erection been? (*Please circle one number*).
   (1) Very poor to none
   (2) Poor
   (3) Fair
   (4) Good
   (5) Very good/Excellent

9. **During the past month**, how often have you experienced a problem remembering something that you thought you knew well? (*Please circle one number*).
   (1) More than once a day
   (2) About once a day
   (3) More than once a week
   (4) About once a week
   (5) Rarely or never

10. During the past month, how often have you felt depressed? (*Please circle one number*).
    (1) More than once a day
    (2) About once a day
    (3) More than once a week
    (4) About once a week
    (5) Rarely or never

11. During the past month, how often have you felt a lack of energy? (*Please circle one number*).
    (1) More than once a day
    (2) About once a day
    (3) More than once a week
    (4) About once a week
    (5) Rarely or never

## Physical Side Effects: Essentials

The physical side effects of ADT can be divided into two major categories: (a) those that impact how your body feels (e.g., hot flashes, loss of muscle strength, fatigue) and (b) those that impact how your body appears (e.g., loss of body hair, gynecomastia, genital shrinkage). Weight gain affects both how your body looks and feels. All of these changes can affect both the patient and his loved ones emotionally. Most patients are likely to experience some, but not necessarily all, side effects.

From a medical perspective, the side effects of greatest concern are those that affect your overall physical health, such as weight gain and bone loss.

Being inactive and overweight increases the risk of other serious illnesses, such as diabetes and cardiovascular disease (leading to heart attack or stroke). Bone loss in turn increases the risk of fracture. You should be aware of these concerns and engage in activities and treatments that can help limit the negative impact of ADT on your overall health.

Exercise and a proper diet are ways to deal with potentially serious complications of ADT. Together they are proven to maintain good health and overall quality of life for patients on ADT. We strongly urge you to incorporate an exercise program into your normal weekly routines *before* you experience the full impact of ADT.

The side effects of ADT can interact with one another. For example, hot flashes that disrupt your sleep can make you tired and less motivated to exercise. But by not exercising you can gain weight, lose bone density, and increase your risk of other serious illnesses.

The side effects that alter male appearance (e.g., gynecomastia, loss of body hair) tend to feminize the body. Patients on ADT do not lose facial hair nor does the pitch of the voice change noticeably; thus, these physical changes do not substantially alter key markers of the male sex. However, you may be understandably distressed by these changes. If you are having difficulty coping with changes in your appearance, consider seeking the help of a professional counselor. Another key to success is to keep communication open with your partner, supportive family members and friends, and, most importantly, with your doctor. Open communication helps to facilitate adaptation to any ADT-related changes.

## Moving Forward: Questions for Discussion

Here are a few questions to help you think about what you learned in this chapter and how it may affect you. Encourage your partner or loved ones to answer these questions too, and discuss your answers with one another. Writing out your answers, and any other questions that may arise from thinking about these topics, is also recommended.

- Of all the physical side effects, the ones I am most concerned about are …
- The side effects that I think my partner might be most concerned about are …
- What are some of the potential solutions I might be willing to try in order to reduce the impact of that side effect?
- Could it help to talk to members of a support group about ADT or to another patient that has experienced ADT first-hand?
- Am I getting enough physical activity? How can I incorporate exercise (cardio, strength training, and flexibility) into my daily life?
- What things can I ask my partner or friends to help me with, in adjusting to the physical side effects of ADT?

**NOTES:**

_____

_____

_____

_____

_____

_____

_____

_____

_____

_____

_____

_____

_____

_____

_____

_____

# 3

# Exercise

---

Men on ADT often gain weight and at the same time experience a decrease in muscle mass, bone density, strength, and overall energy levels. These can contribute to a decreased sense of well-being and quality of life. These side effects persist throughout the course of ADT, which may be for many years, and they often continue after ADT is discontinued. *Regular exercise is the single most important lifestyle factor* that can minimize the negative effects of ADT and help to maintain or recover overall quality of life.

Men on ADT gain numerous health benefits from exercising, no matter what type of exercise is performed. In addition to the positive physical effects of exercising, there are other positive effects on psychological well-being, including reduced fatigue and improved quality of life.

---

*I should have worked against the fatigue by making a daily practice of some type of active exercise, be it a daily, long walk, routine stretching and loosening exercises, etc., but at least something planned. I only continued the routine of most retired men with my only exercise being work around the house, shopping, and the like. I believe that a regular exercise plan and the right mental outlook can counter the effects of fatigue and of muscle loss.*

—Charles (Chuck) Maack, prostate cancer survivor and patient advocate

---

## Exercising Safely

There are several things to consider before beginning an exercise program to ensure that it is undertaken safely and effectively. Here is a list of general safety guidelines that pertain to most endurance/aerobic and resistance training activities:

- Discuss your exercise intentions with your doctor.
- Ask an exercise professional to show you how to safely perform the exercises you plan to do.
- Train with a friend or partner if you are attempting something that may have risks.
- Train in comfortable clothing: running shoes, shorts or track pants, a T-shirt, or moisture-wicking or dry-fit clothes like those made from merino wool that will keep you cool and dry during tough workouts. Protective equipment, such as a helmet, should be worn during any activity that could result in a collision or fall.
- Remember to consume water when working out so you don't get dehydrated.
- Some soreness after a workout is normal. Pain in your joints is not normal and can be a sign of injury. If you are experiencing pain or soreness that lasts longer than three to four days, contact your exercise specialist or see your doctor.

### Caution

The goal of exercise in the context of ADT is to maintain healthy fitness levels and body composition. You should be cautioned not to expect improvements, and warned that some may find that they still gain weight and lose stamina and strength despite regular exercise. If this happens, do not assume that your exercise program is useless. Persist! Many men on ADT get discouraged when they either cannot perform at the level they did previously or they put on weight. Men who were fit prior to ADT seem to be at the highest risk for discouragement. Be aware that even if you feel as if you are still gaining weight and losing muscle mass despite exercising, things would likely be worse if you didn't exercise at all.

Some of the side effects of ADT put patients at increased risk of cardiovascular disease and diabetes. As such, a "heart healthy" diet and exercise form a good program for patients on ADT. Current exercise guidelines for all cancer survivors include 150 minutes of moderate to vigorous intensity exercise per week.

The intensity of an exercise program is how hard you are working during the exercise. Some exercise programs suggest a target heart rate when you are exercising. There are ways to calculate target heart rate based on your age and general health status. However, as a simple guideline, it is a good sign if you are exercising hard enough to sweat. Another useful technique to determine the intensity of your workout is the "talk test." If, when you are exercising, you are breathing hard enough to make it difficult to talk, then you are likely exercising at a vigorous intensity. Low- to moderate-intensity activity does not typically interrupt normal speech, so strive for an intensity that approaches this threshold of the "talk test."

You can prevent unnecessary and potentially dangerous increases in blood pressure if you breathe properly during your training exercises. Breathing out (exhaling), should occur during the "work" phase of the exercise (i.e., the lifting phase), while breathing in (inhaling), should occur during the "relaxing" phase of the exercise (i.e., the lowering or recovery phase). Proper breathing follows a simple four-count pattern: lift—count 1, 2, and lower—count 1, 2. Avoid holding your breath while exercising and try to maintain a steady breathing rhythm.

Your physician, an exercise physiologist, a physiotherapist, or certified trainer should be able to help you fine-tune your exercise program. Adapting an exercise program to address the specific side effects of ADT should include the following:

- Warm-up exercises to prepare your body for more rigorous activity and prevent injury.
- Aerobic exercise to address increases in fat and decreases in cardiovascular fitness.
- Resistance training to address loss of muscle and strength, and to recover functional fitness.
- Weight-bearing and balance activities to maintain bone health and prevent fall-related fractures.
- Stretching to prevent injury, improve balance, and increase flexibility.

## Warm-Up Exercises

A warm-up is a brief period of activity at a lower intensity than is typically achieved during the main portion of the workout. The warm-up is intended to prepare the body for more vigorous activity and reduce the risk of an injury. The exercises, which commonly resemble those used in the main activity (i.e., incorporating the same muscles), can become progressively more intense until the exercise intensity zone of the main workout has been achieved. In terms of intensity, you should not be breathing so hard that you cannot easily maintain a conversation during your warm-up.

Always start your training session by warming up for a few minutes. For example, start your session with stretching and a low-intensity cardiovascular exercise. Consider the following:

- Light stretching or slow movement, including rotating the legs, arms, lower back, and head and neck in circles.
- Walking in place.
- Slow walking.
- Yoga.
- T'ai Chi.

## Aerobic Exercises

Aerobic training, also known as "cardio" training, improves stamina, which is the ability to sustain repeated movements for long durations. Men receiving ADT are at a higher risk of developing cardiovascular disease, obesity, and diabetes. Thirty minutes of aerobic exercises daily is recommended as a key component of maintaining healthy heart and lung function, and potentially reduces the risk of these conditions. You may divide up the time as you wish; three periods of 10 minutes per day are as beneficial as one period of 30 minutes. Start out with exercising for however long you are able, and then try adding 5 minutes to your workouts every week or so. Gradually increase the duration of your cardiovascular exercises up to 30 minutes. Then, increase the intensity of the exercise. Remember the goal is eventually to achieve at least 150 minutes of brisk exercise a week.

Below is a list of aerobic exercises:

- Brisk walking (e.g., walking the dog) or running.
- Mall walking in the winter.
- Stair climbing. (*Note:* Going down stairs can be a little harder on your joints than going up them. If you enjoy climbing stairs, you may want to consider going up one or more flights of stairs and taking the elevator or escalator down.)
- Aqua fitness.
- Dance.
- Rowing.
- Skating.
- Cycling (on either a stationary bike or a road bike).

In many cases, you can listen to music or even watch television while exercising to make the experience more enjoyable.

Consider using a pedometer to keep track of your activity from week-to-week. A pedometer is a movement detector that counts every step you take. It should be clipped to your belt or waistband, midway between your navel and your hip (in line with your kneecap). Using it will allow you to challenge yourself and to observe your progress. There are also now many pedometer "apps" that allow you to use a smart phone as a pedometer.

Also, note that there have been studies done comparing normal walking and brisk walking (i.e., low vs. moderate intensity). Results strongly suggest that the health benefits are much greater with brisk walking.

## Resistance Training

*Resistance training*, also known as *strength training* or *weight lifting*, is the most popular method of building strong, healthy muscles. Safety is a major concern and you should consult with an exercise professional before starting a resistance training program. Resistance training can occur in a variety of ways both with and without equipment.

Since ADT can significantly reduce muscle mass and strength, it is very important that any resistance training program start slowly and progress in resistance. For many exercises your body weight may be enough; while for others it may be beneficial to use free weights or elastic bands. To determine a good workload, do 12 repetitions. The first repetitions should be done quite easily. The last ones (11th and 12th) should be difficult but not impossible. When you are able to do 12 repetitions easily, add another set of 12. We recommend resistance training at least three times per week.

Resistance exercises should work the following muscles:

| Upper Body | Lower Body |
|---|---|
| Pectorals (e.g., push-ups) | Buttocks (e.g., squats, climbing stairs) |
| Shoulders (e.g., shoulder presses) | Quadriceps (e.g., squats) |
| Abdominals (e.g., crunches) | Calves (e.g., leg lifts) |
| Biceps (e.g., bicep curls) | Hamstrings (e.g., squats, climbing stairs) |
| Triceps (e.g., tricep dips) | |

Having the correct posture during your muscular workout is very important in order to prevent injuries. If you are new to these types of exercises, we recommend that you review your exercise program with a fitness instructor or exercise specialist.

Resistance bands, free weights (e.g., barbells, dumbbells), and weight lifting machines are often used for this type of training but are not absolutely necessary. Exercises such as push-ups, leg raises, and abdominal crunches are also useful at building muscle and strength.

## Weight-Bearing Activities

ADT can reduce bone strength, making bones more susceptible to fracture. Two approaches are generally pursued when trying to prevent a fracture: (a) improve bone health and (b) reduce the risk of falls. To achieve these, a comprehensive exercise program should include weight-bearing activities, which promote bone strength as well as balance exercises to prevent falls. Weight-bearing activities promote bone maintenance and development. They include any activity that involves being upright and supporting your weight with your legs. The most common weight-bearing activities are:

- Walking and running.
- Golf, squash, and tennis.
- Skipping.

## Balance Exercises

One of the most important benefits of a regular exercise program is the maintenance of good balance and the resultant reduction in the risk of falls. Your program could incorporate activities specifically designed to maintain and improve balance such as:

- Walking on a line (heel to toe) or on your toes.
- Balancing on one foot.
- Walking backwards or sideways.
- Yoga.

*Note:* These exercises do put you at a risk of a fall, therefore they should first be attempted near a chair or railing that you can hold on to if you start to fall.

## Winding Down

After your workout, give your body a few minutes to relax and wind down. Take advantage of this time to do some stretching. We recommend that you maintain a stretch position for 20 to 30 seconds. You should feel a slight discomfort due to the stretching, but no pain. Repeat each movement a couple of times. Make sure you stretch both sides of your body. Breathe normally without holding your breath. Each stretching movement should be done slowly and gently, and without bouncing.

## Making the Decision to Exercise

### Habit and Reason

A useful tool to help you make the decision to exercise is the Pros/Cons table found on the next page. The table is designed to help you recognize motivations for making changes, but also to increase awareness of the reasons why you may be hesitant to change. Filling in this table can help you to identify barriers that may get in the way of you making changes. Recognizing barriers is the first step to overcoming them.

You have an excellent reason, or a "strong pro," to include exercise in your daily routine, and that is *managing the possible side effects of ADT*! The problem with changing our exercise habits or beginning new ones is that in most cases our physical activity has remained similar for many years and has become cemented in routine and habit. Without thinking about it, we drive to work, we take the elevator, and we sit in front of screens (TV and computers) for many hours each day. And we "accept" that our days are too full for much else. This behavior, termed the "mechanics of habit," needs to be interrupted or broken. One effective way to do this is to examine your reasons for letting everything else in your day take precedent over exercise and your overall health. Examining these reasons and questioning their validity will sharpen your awareness of your sedentary routine and help you to break free of habits that promote reduced physical activity.

We recommend to everyone the 10-minute video *23 and 1/2 Hours: What Is the Single Best Thing We Can Do for Our Health?* (www.youtube.com/watch?v=aUaInS6HIGo). As the video suggests, limit your daily activities (work, sleep, TV, etc.) to 23½ hours a day and use the remaining half hour to exercise.

### Activity: Pros/Cons Table

Your strong reason for exercising, managing the possible side effects of ADT, is likely one of the things you would list in the pros column of a Pros/Cons table. We will always have reasons both for and against making a change in our behavior. This specific pro gives you a head start in overcoming the cons, so start by placing it at the top of your pros list. Be honest with yourself and spend the same time and energy working on the cons as you do on the pros.

**Example:**

|  | PROS | CONS |
|---|---|---|
| **MAKING THE CHANGE:**<br>Exercising | • Reduce the amount of weight I might gain<br><br>• Prevent loss of physical stamina<br><br>• Manage fatigue | • Requires significant planning and effort<br><br>• I will have to reprioritize my schedule so I find time to spend exercising |
| **STAYING THE SAME:**<br>Not exercising | • Easier to just carry on the way I am | • My fatigue may continue to get worse<br><br>• I will feel bad about myself for being unfit |

Try it for yourself. There is an additional blank copy of this table in the Appendix on page 123.

|  | PROS | CONS |
|---|---|---|
| **MAKING THE CHANGE:** |  |  |
| **STAYING THE SAME:** |  |  |

This sounds tedious, but it works. The more the pros outweigh the cons, the stronger your reasons to exercise, which translates into making exercise personally relevant for you. If you find a lot of reasons in your cons list, you may wish to consider another method of achieving your goal.

After you have recorded your pros and cons, see which column has more responses. If your pros of exercising are stronger than your cons, or if there are more of them, then, technically speaking, you've decided that a healthy exercise change is worth it. Keep this list handy while you embark on the next step—starting your exercise program.

### Activity: Identifying and Overcoming Barriers to Starting and Maintaining an Exercise Program

**I feel *too* tired.** When we feel fatigued our instinct is to rest. Those who are struggling with fatigue may worry that they won't have the energy to do their usual activities if they spend energy exercising. You do need to rest, but resting too much can lead to muscle deconditioning, which will in turn lead to more fatigue.

**I don't have the willpower.** You *do* have the willpower; you simply need to find a way to unleash this power! You are prepared. You have the main ingredients to a successful exercise program. Consider this, how often do you dread the thought of something you enjoy? Probably, quite rarely (or never). So if you can find the fun in your activity, it will ensure that your willpower can be realized. Think of ways to integrate things you enjoy while exercising, like music, your friends/family, a television show, or an environment that is relaxing (e.g., park) or stimulating (e.g., gym) for you.

**It's not the right time.** There's no perfect time. Now may be as good a time as any. There will always be some stress in your life. There will always be distractions. You can make progress now.

**My life is all wrong. This little change isn't going to make a difference.** Just the opposite. You've got to start somewhere. If you're sure this is the right place to start, and that you're going in the right direction, then you are already turning wrongs into rights.

**I have aches and/or pain that limits how I can exercise.** We all have certain aches and pains that make some exercises uncomfortable or possibly painful. It's important to avoid exercises that cause pain. If the pain persists when you are not exercising, you should consult your physician. For any aches and pains that you have that may limit your activities, consider alternate forms of exercise. For example, if walking bothers your knees, try cycling, swimming, or using an elliptical machine. Or, if certain resistance training exercises cause discomfort in your back or shoulders, speak with an exercise specialist for adjustments to these exercises so they suit your body better.

**Other barrier and ways to address or challenge this barrier:**

_____

_____

_____

## Activity: Matching Meaning and Change
## Using Self-Statements

Changing behavior is a challenge. We are forced to ignore old comfortable patterns of behavior and embrace new, less familiar ones. A lot is happening at once. People face behavioral change on a moment-by-moment, situation-by-situation basis. This step-by-step process is necessary in the gentle acquisition of change. However, in the early stages of change, people can lose track of why they decided to change in the first place. In their daily "struggles," the meaning of the change can be lost. Ironically, your reasons for initiating change are probably more important early in the change process than at any other time.

A simple method of maintaining your awareness of why you decided to change is the use of "self-statements." Consider the Pros/Cons table you completed in Chapter 2 (p. 21). Write down your most meaningful pros below. These are your "meaning self-statements." If you ever feel that things are not progressing as quickly as you want, or you feel that you are slipping, read these self-statements to reinforce the meaning of your change.

**Meaning Self-Statements:**

1. _____

_____

_____

2. _____

_____

_____

3. _____

_____

_____

## Preparing to Successfully Begin Exercising

Thinking is the first essential step, but thinking is not doing. Are you ready to move from thinking about it to actively planning for it? Thorough preparation is key to successfully begin exercising. These questions will assist you in developing your Action Plan.

### Make an Action Plan

It is important to know when, where, and with whom you plan to exercise, and what type of exercise(s) you will perform.

### What I Plan to Do:

It is important to choose exercise activities that you believe will benefit your health (i.e., exercises you have confidence in) and that you believe you can maintain over time (i.e., exercises that you have confidence you can perform). There are a wide variety of exercises available to choose from, so take your time. You may want to test out different ones to see which exercises suit you best. To successfully challenge the effects of ADT, choose an exercise or two from each of the exercise categories: warm-up, aerobic, resistance, and weight-bearing.

### When I Plan to Do It:

- A time free of stress.
- A time when you can put out some extra effort.
- A time when you will have the support you need.

   Which days of the week work best for you? _____

   What time of the day is most suitable for you?_____

   How long do you want to exercise during each session?_____

*Note:* You should allow specific muscle groups 48 hours of rest in between each resistance workout to allow for proper healing. Also, remember to wait at least one hour after a meal before exercising.

### Where I Plan to Do It:

- Inside or outside? Adapt your program to the season.
- *Indoor*—in your home, at a gym, in a "rehab" center or hospital, or in a peer support community center. Remember, you can also do many exercises in your home with a few inexpensive pieces of equipment such as resistance bands and a stability or exercise ball.
- *Outdoor*—in a park, on a cycling trail, at a resort or club, or a walking/ running circuit in your neighborhood.

   Be as specific as possible about where you plan to exercise:

_____

_____

**Who I Might Do It With:**

- Usually teaming up with someone helps with sticking to a program. By holding each other accountable, you'll both benefit from increased exercise.
- If you have a partner, start with that individual. There are few better ways to ensure ongoing success than engaging your partner to exercise with you.
- Talk to your friends and neighbors to find out what type of exercise they do and see if you can join them.

  Is there a cancer-specific exercise group that you can join?_____

  _____

- Sometimes having the support of others going through a similar experience can be very positive.

  Who do you plan to exercise with? Or are you better off exercising on your own?_____

  _____

### Activity: Action Plan · · · · · · · · · · · · · · · · · · · ·

Much of the information gathered in the previous pages (what, where, when, with whom) can be summarized using an Action Plan. See below for an example. Remember that it is best to start small with something manageable (e.g., go to the gym twice a week) before you take on larger scale goals (e.g., go to the gym every day).

### Action Plan Example: Start Walking Routinely

**What I plan to do:** walk for 15 minutes or more, three times a week

**When I plan to do it:** Monday, Wednesday, and Friday after work

**Who I might do it with:** with my partner and/or with my dog

**Why my plan is important:** to help control my health risks and reduce fatigue

**Where I plan to do it:** around my neighborhood

**What might get in the way?** poor weather

**How I will address what might get in the way:** I will go to the mall to walk

Try it yourself. An additional copy is located in the Appendix on page 124. It helps to be as specific as possible when you are making your Action Plan.

**Action plan:** _____

What I plan to do: _____

_____

When I plan to do it: _____

_____

Who I might do it with: _____

_____

Why my plan is important: _____

_____

Where I plan to do it: _____

_____

What might get in the way? _____

_____

How I will address what might get in the way: _____

_____

Hang your Action Plan somewhere where you will see it every day, like next to your bathroom mirror, to remind yourself of your commitment to exercise.

## Activity: Goal Setting and Confidence

You have identified what type of exercise(s) you plan to do. Now, in order to support your goal, it can be helpful to ask yourself how confident you are that you can be successful in making this change. First, write down your goal.

**Goal 1:** _____
   (e.g., Warm-up, weight-bearing, resistance, aerobic, wind down)

i) Rate how confident you feel that you'll achieve your exercise goal:
   1     2     3     4     5     6     7     8     9     10
   Not confident                                    Very confident

ii) Rate how motivated you are to accomplish your exercise goal:
   1     2     3     4     5     6     7     8     9     10
   Not motivated                                    Very motivated

iii) Rate how likely you are to actually carry out your exercise goal:
   1     2     3     4     5     6     7     8     9     10
   Not likely                                        Very likely

**Goal 2:** _____
   (e.g., weight-bearing, resistance, aerobic)

i)  Rate how confident you feel that you'll achieve your exercise goal:
    1      2      3      4      5      6      7      8      9      10
    Not confident                                    Very confident

ii) Rate how motivated you are to accomplish your exercise goal:
    1      2      3      4      5      6      7      8      9      10
    Not motivated                                    Very motivated

iii) Rate how likely you are to actually carry out your exercise goal:
    1      2      3      4      5      6      7      8      9      10
    Not likely                                       Very likely

**A note about confidence—it counts!** Behavioral science research has determined that one's level of confidence in embarking on a health-related change is the strongest predictor of success.

- Any exercise recommendation that you choose with a confidence rating of less than 7 out of 10 may represent your Achilles' heel. Knowing this can help you realize the extra attention and effort that a particular exercise recommendation may require. We suggest that you do not take on more than two recommendations with a confidence rating lower than 7.
- If your motivation level is low, it may be a good time to go back and reexamine what you put in the Pros/Cons table.
- If you do not think you are likely to carry out your exercise goal, it may be better to select a different goal, one that you are more likely to carry out. Small successes can act as momentum, whereas aiming too high can act as a roadblock. Start small with goals that you are confident you can achieve. For example, start taking the stairs instead of the elevator, or stand up and do some stretching every 30 minutes during your workday.

### Maintaining Your Motivation

You have made your change and are exercising regularly. Congratulations! You may be finding your new exercise routine to be no big deal or still a challenge. Either way, you have taken an important step. Getting to the point of exercising regularly is a long and difficult process, and you have done it. This section offers some tips to help you maintain your exercise regimen once you have started.

### Managing Lapses and Relapses

A lapse differs from a relapse in both *frequency* and *duration*. A *lapse* is a single instance of failing to stick to your exercise plan; a *relapse* is a series of lapses in succession. Lapses last only as long as it takes to deviate from your exercise plan, for example, the time it takes to miss a planned exercise session. Relapses are lapses repeated and prolonged; that is, missing exercise sessions again and again, sometimes for a short duration (e.g., one week while on vacation), but usually over much longer periods.

Most people experience lapses and relapses when they try to make a significant healthy change such as maintaining an exercise program. They are a normal and expected part of real life. How those lapses are managed determines how seriously they threaten long-term change. You will experience a lapse or relapse at some point; just remember that exercising regularly is a step-by-step, day-by-day process. You can easily miss a step or two, or day or two, and lose enthusiasm. The key is to turn around the lapse or relapse quickly by restarting your exercises as soon as possible. A lapse or relapse is a slip, and a slip is not failure. Decisive action and careful planning have enabled you to build a foundation for exercising. Upon a lapse or relapse, we suggest you return to this foundation and review your reasons and plans for exercising (the Pros/Cons table), as well as your methods for handling hard times. Use this reexamination to challenge the lapse or relapse. Managing these temporary setbacks is not that different than making the original commitment to change. But remember, the longer the relapse, the more vulnerable your commitment to exercise.

### Reward Yourself

Rewarding yourself is an art. So do it artfully. Try to reward yourself consistently. Don't worry about being too conventional and don't wait until the victory is won. Rewarding yourself amid the struggle is more important. During the first two weeks of exercising, try rewarding yourself a little each day. A good reward might be sleeping in an extra 10 minutes, new exercise apparel, some new music to listen to while you exercise, watching a movie, or making time to meet with friends. It doesn't have to take long and it need not be expensive. Choose a reward that inspires you to exercise and it can help you stay on track.

Some rewards, however, can actually deter you from your overall fitness goals. Often food is used as a reward. It is okay to treat yourself with a "not-so-healthy-snack"—occasionally! If having a food reward encourages you to exercise, then it's a great idea. Regardless of the calorie count, you are exercising and still improving cardiovascular fitness! It may be a helpful point of awareness to think about it this way: A small bag (1.69 oz package; 1.7 oz = ~48 g) of M&M's is a nice reward; however, it is 240 calories. If you want to balance your calorie intake, 30 minutes on the treadmill will burn off those calories.

Another "reward" that is often implemented is a decrease in nonexercise physical activity. For example, if you had a great workout, you might feel like avoiding the stairs that you usually take to your apartment or office. By avoiding these other daily activities you are simply trading one healthy behavior for another, resulting in less net benefit. Try to maintain your daily, nonexercise physical activities. Compensating for healthy behaviors with unhealthy ones too frequently can undermine your progress. So again, give yourself a treat when you've done a good job with your exercise, but too many treats (or the wrong treats) may in fact set you back.

### Support

Research has shown that social support contributes to healthy change. In study after study, support has made a major difference in successful exercising, especially if your spouse/partner or a close friend is also participating in exercising. A joint effort to exercise regularly promotes mutual encouragement.

Providing support to your significant other for exercise, and vice versa, may be the best support you can provide.

The key ingredients of "precise support" are threefold:

- *Timing:* It must be there *when* a person needs it.
- *Focus:* It must be focused *where* a person needs it—emotionally, practically, and so on.
- *Expression:* It must be expressed in the specific way that best motivates the individual to achieve his or her goal.

## Exercise: Essentials

Exercise is one of the most important things you can do to manage ADT side effects. Men on ADT often gain weight as fat, at the same time experiencing a decrease in muscle mass, bone density, strength, and overall energy levels. Exercise can help manage all of these side effects.

We discussed the rationale for beginning an exercise program and gave recommendations for creating one that works best for you. We also acknowledged that maintaining an exercise program over the long-term can be difficult and provided tips on making exercise safe and enjoyable, as well as strategies that will help you overcome challenges that may arise.

Successful change lies in decision making, planning, initiating, trial and error, and maintaining—all leading to confidence in ongoing change. As you continue your journey toward ongoing regular exercise, increased confidence will lead to an increase in your success, overcoming lapses and relapses quickly. In time, this feedback loop from action to confidence to action again will result in the integration of exercise into your everyday life. Incorporating regular exercise into your routine may very well be the single most important thing you do to maintain a good quality of life while on ADT.

### Moving Forward: Questions for Discussion

- What physical activities do I enjoy most?
- Who would I enjoy exercising with?
- What are the three most important reasons for me to exercise?
- What time of the day would I feel most comfortable and motivated to exercise?
- I have a few lingering aches and pains or injuries, such as ...
  How will I adapt my physical activities to prevent them from being aggravated?
- What equipment or supplies do I require to exercise effectively, and where can I access them?
- What barriers to exercise can I anticipate encountering as I begin to try to maintain an exercise program? How will I address them?
- Three specific goals I have at the end of six weeks of exercise are ...
- To reward myself for exercise, I will ...

**NOTES:**

_____

_____

_____

_____

_____

_____

_____

_____

_____

# 4

# Healthy Eating

When you are on ADT, you may experience common side effects such as a loss of muscle mass and weight gained as fat mainly at your waistline. Men treated with ADT are also at increased risk of osteoporosis, diabetes, and cardiovascular problems. Over time, ADT causes decreases in bone mineral density, increased body weight, poor blood sugar regulation, and raised cholesterol and triglycerides that can all contribute to these risks. Fortunately, eating healthy can help you to manage your weight and reduce these risk factors.

As a general rule, eating healthy involves consuming lots of fruits, vegetables, and lean protein. Eating healthy also means eating fresh food as much as possible. Foods that have been processed often contain high amounts of salt, sugar, preservatives, and unhealthy fats. Processed foods also tend to be lower in nutrition and higher in calories.

**RECOMMENDATIONS:**
- Eat less saturated and trans fats.
- Eat more high-fiber foods (e.g., whole grains, vegetables, nuts, and fruits).
- Limit salt and sugar intake.
- Eat more white meat (e.g., fish, chicken) than red meat (e.g., beef, pork, and lamb).
- Eat less processed and junk foods.

## Reading Food Labels

Most packaged foods in the United States and Canada have mandatory nutrition labeling. Read the labels carefully and make an effort to eat food with the highest nutritional content. The values on most labels are based on a diet of 2,000 calories (cal) per day. Look for foods or beverages high in nutrients such as calcium, vitamin C, vitamin A, thiamin, niacin, and fiber. Also check the amounts of fat (saturated and trans fat), cholesterol, sugar, and sodium—and limit these nutrients. Remember to look at the serving size and the total number of calories, and compare this to the portion you actually eat. The Percent Daily Value (%DV) on the Nutrition Facts table provides information on calories and 13 nutrients. This can be used to compare products and make a healthier choice. It helps to know what is the recommended daily allowance (RDA) for each nutrient that is discussed further below. A quick rule for using the %DV is that 5% or less is a small amount of a nutrient in an overall day, and 20% or higher is a lot for a single food in a day.

> The U.S. Department of Health & Human Services has more information regarding labels, including some helpful graphics. This can be accessed on their website (www.fda.gov) under the "Food" tab.

## Fats

Fats provide energy and, when stored as body fat, help to keep your body warm. Fats also provide the building materials for cells and some hormones, and they help the body absorb some vitamins. Your body needs fat to function, but moderation is important. Too much fat can be damaging to your health. Eating a high-fat diet increases your risk of obesity and related health problems, such as heart disease and diabetes. Because these are the same health risks men experience on ADT, combining a high-fat diet with ADT will make you more susceptible to these health problems.

Fats are classified into two groups:

1. *Unsaturated fats* are generally considered to be the "healthy" fats. They are categorized as either *monounsaturated* (found in olive and canola oils, avocados, and most nuts) or *polyunsaturated* (found in vegetable oils, meat products, and fish). There are some types of polyunsaturated fatty acids that your body cannot produce, but still needs. These are considered "essential" fatty acids and must be obtained from your diet. Linoleic acid (omega-6; LA), and alpha-linolenic acid (omega-3; ALA) are two polyunsaturated fatty acids that are considered "essential." They should be consumed regularly, but in moderation. To learn more about omega fatty acids, see pages 54 to 56.

2. *Saturated fats* are considered to be the "less healthy" fats. Although it is unrealistic to avoid all saturated fats, they should be limited as much as possible. Saturated fats are solid at room temperature. Most of the saturated fats in our diet come from animal products, such as meat and dairy.

Trans fats are a type of unsaturated fat, but they are an exception to the "healthy" rule as they are processed in the body similarly to saturated fats. Trans fats are present naturally in small quantities in foods such as meat and dairy, but in Western diets most trans fats come from processed foods during a process called *hydrogenation*. This process turns oils into semisolid products, including partially hydrogenated oils such as vegetable shortening and some types of margarine. Hydrogenation makes food products last longer, but it also makes trans fats especially harmful. Other foods containing trans fats include potato chips, chocolate bars, and many foods made from or fried in hydrogenated fat. When shopping, it is recommended to read the labels to determine the amount of trans fats in the products you buy, and aim to pick foods with no (or limited) trans fats in them.

Dietary fats are a part of the building blocks of androgens. There is some evidence that high-fat diets can raise androgen levels. For example, vegetarians (who often consume less dietary fat) tend to have lower levels of testosterone than meat eaters. One theory under investigation is whether men with prostate cancer may benefit from a diet lower in fat and cholesterol aimed at decreasing testosterone. The goal of reducing testosterone is similar to treatment with ADT, which attempts to "starve" prostate cancer cells of testosterone.

**RECOMMENDATIONS:**

- Start by cutting back on fried and processed foods.
- Eat smaller (palm-sized) portions of meat, especially red meat.
- When preparing poultry or other meats, remove the skin and trim off excess fat.
- If you fry your meat, remember to drain the fat from the pan before adding sauces.
- Stir-frying, sautéing, baking, or grilling your food are all better options than frying or deep-frying.
- Cut down on butter, margarine, oils, sauces, gravy, and cream.
- Aim to eat more fruits and vegetables that are naturally lower in fat.
- Focus on quality, also keeping in mind the amount that you eat.
- Choose plant-based fats such as olive, safflower, canola, or sesame oils, which have greater health benefits.

Be aware of what you're eating—choose lower fat foods when you shop for groceries. When choosing low-fat items, some are better in nutritional value than others. Lower fat dairy products are a good choice because only the fat is reduced. However, be mindful that lower fat foods may replace the fat with sugar, so aim for foods with a lower calorie count.

Pretty soon, making healthier choices will become a habit.

## Protein

Our bodies need protein to build tissue for growth and repair. The protein in our diets comes from two sources: animals and plants. Animal sources of protein include red meats (e.g., beef, pork, and lamb), white meats (e.g., poultry, fish), and dairy products. Red and white meat are protein rich, and red meat may provide slight added benefits like vitamin $B_{12}$ and iron. Despite these benefits, there are a few things you need to consider when purchasing them.

Western diets typically include too much animal protein and not enough vegetables, fruits, and legumes. Most cuts of red meat are also high in fat, and processed meats (e.g., bacon, deli meats) are often also high in salt, fat, and preservatives. White meat is typically a better healthy choice compared to red meat. Furthermore, meat cooked at high temperatures that results in charring can burn off protein and form cancer-causing products.

Fish is a "heart-healthier" and leaner source of protein because most types are naturally low in fat. Be careful, though—canned fish packed in oil can be high in fat. Also, frying any type of fish may increase the amount of unhealthy fat you are ingesting. Steaming or broiling is a better option.

Milk and dairy products can also be very high in fat, particularly saturated fat. When eating dairy, it is recommended that you opt for lower fat choices (i.e., skim or 1% milks, low-fat cheeses, and yogurts), and look for dairy products that don't have a lot of added sugars.

The following table describes various sources of protein.

| Meat or Meat Alternative | Serving Size or Amount |
|---|---|
| Cooked fish, shellfish, poultry, or lean meat (beef, pork, lamb) | 2 1/2 oz (75 g) or 1/2 cup (125 mL) or the size of a deck of playing cards |
| Cooked beans, peas, lentils, or tofu | 3/4 cup (175 mL) |
| Nuts or seeds (shelled) | 1/4 cup (60 mL) |
| Peanut butter or other nut butters | 2 tbsp (30 mL) |
| Eggs | 2 eggs |

Based on the *Dietary Reference Intakes for Americans and Canadians*, it is recommended that adults consume 0.8 g of protein per kg of body weight. On average that means a daily intake of 46 g of protein for women and 56 g for men.

A strategy for finding the right fat–protein balance is to focus on plant protein. Plants that provide protein are typically rich in vitamins and minerals, low in fat and sodium, plus they provide fiber. Unlike meat, plant proteins are high in carbohydrates (the "complex" or starchy type; see table below). The richest sources of plant protein are legumes, such as dried peas (e.g., split peas) and beans (e.g., kidney, chickpea).

Include a variety of plant protein sources in your daily diet. The following table gives you an idea of some plant protein sources:

| Legumes | Grain | Nuts and Seeds |
|---|---|---|
| Soybeans/soy products | Barley | Almonds |
| Peanuts | Bulgur | Walnuts |
| Chickpeas | Couscous | Cashews |
| Lentils | Oats | Chestnuts |
| Split peas | Rice | Pecans |
| Kidney beans | Wheat | Pumpkin seeds |
| Pinto beans | Rye | Sesame seeds |
| Fava beans | | Quinoa |

Legumes, nuts, and seeds are the best sources of plant protein. Grains provide a small amount of protein to a diet, particularly for vegetarians. Quinoa, which is sometimes eaten in similar ways to a grain, is actually a seed and is rich in protein.

Plant foods are high in fiber and you may experience gastrointestinal problems if you increase your consumption too quickly. Try introducing plant protein gradually into your diet, and drink water with your meals.

### RECOMMENDATIONS:

- Replace protein foods that are higher in fat, preservatives, and salt with those that are lower.
- Substitute seafood for red meat at least once a week.
- Eat a variety of protein foods, which include seafood, lean meat and poultry, eggs, beans and peas, soy products, and unsalted nuts and seeds.
- Choose low-fat or fat-free milk and milk products, such as milk, yogurt, and cheese.

## Carbohydrates

Carbohydrates are a source of energy. Although they often get a bad reputation for being "fattening," in reality, carbohydrates have fewer calories (or food energy) per gram than fats (4 cal compared with 9 cal). Carbohydrates are classified as simple or complex, based on the size of the molecules.

*Simple carbohydrates* are sugars and can be monosaccharides (glucose, fructose, galactose) or disaccharides (maltose, sucrose, lactose). They are absorbed quickly into the body, raising blood sugar, and are considered "fast" energy. Foods such as honey, molasses, white sugar, brown sugar, raw sugar, and maple and corn syrups are similar in nutritional value and high in simple carbohydrates.

*Complex carbohydrates* are polysaccharides, sometimes called *starches* and *fiber*. Polysaccharides are digested and absorbed slower than simple carbohydrates, but are also eventually broken down into sugars. Starches are present in grains, legumes, and root vegetables (e.g., potatoes and yams).

Fiber is found only in plant foods, such as fruits and vegetables, grains, and legumes. It is the indigestible part of the plant. Fiber nevertheless has many benefits in the digestion of foods in general. Aim for at least 25 grams of fiber daily. Plant foods that are rich in fiber are also a good source of carbohydrates.

### RECOMMENDATIONS:

- Eat whole foods rich in complex carbohydrates, such as whole grains, legumes, fruits, and vegetables as part of your balanced diet.
- Limit "refined" carbohydrates found in starchy and sugary processed foods. The processing lowers their nutritional value.
- Limit products with added sugar. They have extra calories without any other nutritional benefit.

### Determining Your Current BMI

BMI stands for *body mass index*. This measure is a tool that can help determine if you are presently at a healthy weight for your height. You can ask your local gym or your family doctor to help you determine your BMI. The BMI is a generalization of body type; it does not differentiate fat weight from fat-free weight (muscle or bone). If you are not convinced your BMI is accurate, having your body fat percentage and/or waist-to-hip ratio measured may help to better determine your healthy weight range.

If you would like to determine your BMI on your own, you can use the following formulas:

*English*: BMI = weight in pounds/(height in inches × height in inches) × 703
*Metric*: BMI = weight in kilograms/(height in meters × height in meters)

Pay special attention to the units in the formula, otherwise the result will not be accurate. There are also many BMI calculators available online.

*Note*: For persons 65 years and older, the "normal" range may begin slightly above BMI 18.5 and extend into the "overweight" range. The BMI may underestimate body fat in older persons.

Below are the different classifications of BMI and their health risks:

| Classification | BMI Category | Risk of Developing Health Problems |
| --- | --- | --- |
| Underweight | <18.5 | Increased |
| Normal weight | 18.5–24.9 | Least |
| Overweight | 25.0–29.9 | Increased |
| Obese | ≥30.0 | High |

Although not as precise as the BMI, measuring one's waist circumference can be a good approximation of where one stands in terms of health risks. The higher the waist circumference is above the population average, the greater are the health risks. In North America, the "cut-off" for what is considered healthy is 40 inches (102 cm) for men and 35 inches (88 cm) for women. Measurements above these values for waist circumference put you at greater risk for developing health problems.

### Estimating Your Nutritional Needs

The Dietary Reference Intakes (in Canada and the United States) currently recommend the following percentages for daily calorie intake:

- *Fat*: 20% to 35% (no more than 10% from saturated sources)
- *Protein*: 10% to 35%
- *Carbohydrate*: 45% to 65%

If you decide to change your diet to meet these recommendations, remember that the goal is to maintain your present calorie (energy) intake, assuming you are at a healthy weight right now. To keep your calories balanced, when you add more of certain types of food to your diet (e.g., complex carbohydrates, such as those in whole grain cereals or breads) you will need to decrease calories from other foods (e.g., saturated fats).

To estimate your daily requirements, decide on a realistic goal for the percentage of fat, protein, and carbohydrates you would like to eat, from within the recommended ranges. Protein, like carbohydrates, has approximately 4 calories per gram. Fats have 9 calories per gram. Alcohol also contributes calories (about 7 cal/g), so don't forget to factor it in, if you drink.

Using an estimated calorie goal based on your activity level, you can calculate the grams of fat, protein, and carbohydrates using the following equation:

[(Calories × Percentage of intake)/Calories per gram of carbohydrate, protein, or fat] = [Daily grams of carbohydrate, protein, or fat]

For example, if you eat about 2,000 calories per day, and you would like to eat 55% of your total calories as carbohydrates, the amount in grams would be calculated as follows:

[(2,000 calories × 0.55)/4 calories per gram] = 275 grams of carbohydrate per day

There is no golden rule to follow when determining your daily calorie intake; it depends on several factors, including your weight, age, sex, and activity level. A typical value for a middle-aged man is about 2,000 to 2,500 calories per day. To estimate your calorie consumption, record what you eat for several days and calculate your average intake. For more precise calculations, consult a dietitian to evaluate your energy requirements.

If you find that you are putting on weight while on ADT, you may need to lower your calorie intake. Remember, if you need to lose weight, for best results you will need to consistently eat less and/or burn off more calories than your body typically needs in a day. You cannot lose weight if you take in more calories than you burn off.

> For more information on nutrition and weight management, help on tracking what you eat, an online BMI calculator, and more, visit www.choosemyplate.gov, a website designed by the U.S. Department of Agriculture. The Academy of Nutrition and Dietetics (www.eatright.org) is also an excellent resource. There are also several "apps" available to help you track your food intake and your physical activity.

## Omega-3 Fatty Acids

Omega-3 fatty acids are important for overall health and are found mainly in fish, seafood, some nuts, seeds, and vegetable oils. There are three types of polyunsaturated omega-3 fatty acids: ALA, eicosapentaenoic acid (EPA), and docosahexaenoic acid (DHA). ALA is called an essential fatty acid because it cannot be formed in the body; it must be acquired through your diet. Rich sources are flaxseed, meats, and cereals. ALA can be converted to EPA and DHA in our bodies, but this process is inefficient; therefore, it is best to include foods rich in all three types of omega-3 fatty acids in your diet. EPA and DHA are found in fatty, cold-water fish such as salmon, herring, mackerel, sardines, bass, and white albacore tuna. Fish are recommended as an excellent source of omega-3 fatty acids.

### Omega-3 Fatty Acid Supplements

Foods are the preferred way to meet daily needs. Foods have a wide range of other vitamins, minerals, fiber, and anticancer compounds not found in supplements and do not have the same risk of possible adverse effects. Although diets rich in ALA have been shown to reduce heart disease in men, the role of omega-3 fatty acids or fish oil supplements (rich in omega-3) in decreasing prostate cancer progression remains unclear. Men with prostate cancer are recommended to eat fish twice per week and include other foods rich in omega-3 fatty acids as part of their daily diet for general health benefits.

Furthermore, there is no evidence to suggest that men already diagnosed with prostate cancer benefit from omega-3 supplements. Men with a family history of stroke or on blood-thinning medications (including aspirin) could, in rare instances, experience negative side effects. If you are thinking of taking a supplement rich in omega-3, you should consult with your physician or a registered dietitian first.

The best food sources of omega-3 include the following:

- Fish and seafood including herring, anchovies, mackerel, sardines, salmon, whitefish, halibut, trout, oysters, Arctic char, cod, tuna, and mussels.
- Some vegetable oils, including flaxseed and canola oil.
- Some plant foods are a rich source (e.g., some nuts and seeds). The best sources are flaxseed (ground), chia and hemp seeds, walnuts, and soy foods including soybeans, edamame, and tofu. Other nuts, such as pecans, also contain omega-3.

*Note:* This list includes food sources and not any supplement sources of omega-3 fatty acids such as fish oils.

In addition, some foods are now fortified with omega-3 fats and therefore become good sources. Foods commonly fortified include some brands of milk, soy beverages, yogurt, and eggs. Check the label!

A limited amount of omega-3 fatty acids are found in grains, such as wheat germ. But otherwise, grains and most vegetables and fruit are *not* good sources.

### RECOMMENDATIONS:

- Get your omega-3 fatty acids from eating fish and other sources, rather than from taking supplements.
- Eating fish even once a week may be enough to reap some positive benefits.
- The RDA for omega-3 fatty acids is 1.6 grams for adult males.

### Omega-6 Fatty Acids

Linoleic acid is a type of essential omega-6 fatty acid and is found in animal fats, nuts, and vegetable oils. It is the most commonly consumed polyunsaturated fatty acid in the Western diet. Because it is so common in popular foods, we often eat more than we need. It is recommended that you try to balance your omega-3 and omega-6 intake by substituting fish for meat at least once a week and choosing oils with less omega-6.

Dietary recommendations for omega-3 and omega-6 are shown in the following table:

| Fatty Acid | Age | General Recommended Daily Intake (g) |
| --- | --- | --- |
| Omega-3 | All ages | 1.6* |
| Omega-6 | 31–50 years | 17 |
| | 51 and older | 14 |

*Up to 10% of daily intake can be consumed as EPA and/or DHA.

### RECOMMENDATIONS:

- Use olive oil or canola oil instead of safflower, sunflower, or soybean oil.
- Remember: A little oil goes a long way.

### Soy

Soy foods are recommended as part of a healthy diet and may have additional benefits for men with prostate cancer. Soy is a great substitute for meat because it is a rich source of protein that is low in saturated fat. It also contains special compounds called isoflavones, which, among other things, may help reduce the risk of prostate cancer progression and reduce your likelihood of developing osteoporosis or cardiovascular disease. Soy-based foods are becoming more popular and are easy to find in grocery stores. However, how beneficial soy is in controlling prostate cancer is still under investigation. Here is a list of common soy foods:

*Tofu* is a semisoft food made from adding mineral salt to soymilk. It is a handy and nutritious substitute for meat. Tofu can be purchased as varying degrees of firmness. The softer form is best for sauces and dips; the denser type for grilling, baking, and stir-frying. Tofu lends itself well to a variety of recipes because it absorbs flavors mixed in with it.

*Soy beverage* is made from ground and cooked soybeans. The soy "milk" is filtered out during this process. It can be used as a dairy substitute, drunk straight from the carton, put on your breakfast cereal, or used in cooking or baking. Soy beverages with the highest nutritional value are those fortified with calcium and vitamin D (check the label) and those made with whole soybean, rather than extracts such as "soy protein isolates." "Plain" or "original" beverages are also best because they contain less added sugars than flavored soy beverages.

*Tempeh*, a textured vegetable protein (TVP) made from cooked and fermented soybeans, like other soy foods, can also be used as a meat substitute. It's high in calcium, iron, zinc, and fiber and, like all plant foods, is cholesterol free. Another TVP, *miso*, is made from fermented soybean paste and is commonly used in soups. Miso contains a lot of salt, though, so it should not be eaten in large quantities.

*Natto*, yet another fermented soy product, has a sticky texture and a distinct smell. It is often served on top of rice.

*Soy powder* is available in different flavors, as flour (whole-ground soy flour is best), granules, or the extracted protein (i.e., "isolate"). Among the soy products, defatted soy flour and soy isolates contain the most protein. Soy powder can be mixed with fruit juices, soy beverage, or skim milk. However, overall, soy foods are preferred over soy powders.

*Soy sauce* and *tamari*: Many types of "soy sauce" aren't made from soybeans at all—they're just colored, flavored, salted water. To get the real benefit of soy, use tamari, which is a fermented brew made from soybeans.

## RECOMMENDATIONS:

- Soy is a rich source of protein, and for maximum health benefits, soy can be used as a meat substitute.
- Adding soy (or any new food) to your diet may cause you to gain a few pounds if there is no reduction in other foods. But soy foods can be used as a substitute for meat and thus can help you to avoid gaining weight. Substituting soy for meat can also improve the quality of fat in your diet by adding healthier plant fats.
- Levels of isoflavones, and the amount of protein, fat, and calcium can differ widely across brands and forms of soy products. Read the labels carefully to assess their nutritional value.
- Choose regular or low-fat varieties. If you are drinking soy as a substitute for milk, select soy beverages fortified with calcium.
- Avoid nonfat soy beverages, since soybeans lose some of their beneficial properties when completely defatted.
- Men on protein-restricted diets for medical reasons (e.g., diabetes, liver or kidney disease) should consult their doctor before adding soy to their diet.

## Vitamin D

Vitamin D increases the body's ability to absorb calcium, which is important for bone health. Vitamin D also plays a role in controlling cell growth. Sunlight triggers the body to produce vitamin D, and is the main source of this nutrient. But sunshine doesn't do this very well for certain populations, such as African American and elderly men, and in areas where sunlight is limited (resulting in low vitamin D levels, at least for periods during the year).

At this time the strongest evidence for vitamin D relates to maintaining bone health. Research into the possible benefits of vitamin D for men with prostate cancer is currently in progress.

### How Do I Get Enough Vitamin D?

A primary food source of vitamin D is fatty fish, but North Americans often do not eat enough fish and may get more of their vitamin D from fortified foods. In Canada, it is mandatory for vitamin D to be added to milk. Other foods, such as margarine, soy and rice beverages, goat's milk, orange juice, and some cereals may also have vitamin D added. In the United States, most milk is voluntarily fortified with 100 IU of vitamin D per cup. The Dietary Reference Intakes for Canadians and Americans recommend a daily vitamin D intake of 600 IU (up to age 70) and up to 800 IU (over age 70) from all sources. At present, the tolerable upper limit (UL) is considered to be 4,000 IU/day (from all sources). You may have noticed that there is a wide range of recommendations for vitamin D from other organizations (generally these recommendations advise from 600 IU up to 2,000 IU per day). The *most* ideal daily dose of vitamin D is an active area of research.

In spring and summer, 15 minutes a day of direct sun exposure without sunscreen in the early morning or late afternoon is adequate for most people to meet the RDA for vitamin D within their own body. With this small amount of exposure, the risk of skin cancer is miniscule.

Finally, as the following table indicates, fish are a good dietary source of vitamin D:

| Type of Fish | Vitamin D (IU/100 g) |
| --- | --- |
| Atlantic cod | 40* |
| Tuna (canned in oil, drained) | 236 |
| Atlantic mackerel | 324* |
| Catfish (wild) | 450* |
| Pacific sardines (canned in tomato sauce, drained) | 480 |
| Greenland halibut | 540* |
| Sockeye salmon (canned, drained) | 763 |
| Atlantic herring | 1,465* |

*IU calculated for cooked fish based on raw weights.

## Calcium

Calcium is an important mineral, which helps to build and maintain strong bones. The RDA is 1,000 to 1,200 mg. Despite these benefits, recent studies have found a possible association between *excessive* calcium intake and prostate cancer. It is possible to get too much calcium. The UL for calcium is 2,500 mg (under age 50) and 2,000 mg (over age 50). Research has shown that men who consume 2,000 mg or more of calcium per day (from a combination of diet and supplements) experience an elevated risk of advanced and metastatic disease. Another important side effect of too much calcium is the risk of kidney stones.

This does not mean that men should stop eating dairy or other calcium-rich foods; calcium intake within the RDA has not been linked to prostate cancer. Men with prostate cancer should try to achieve the RDA through diet. It is best not to exceed 1,200 mg of calcium per day (from all sources, diet and supplements), unless specifically advised by your physician.

### Calcium in Your Diet

An adult man (19–70 years old) should consume 1,000 mg of calcium a day. If you are age 70 or older you should consume 1,200 mg per day. This is particularly important for men on long-term ADT, because of the increased risk of osteoporosis associated with this treatment. If you follow the recommendations here, you will likely meet your daily need.

You can access a useful tool for calculating your calcium intake at Osteoporosis Canada's website (www.osteoporosis.ca/osteoporosis-and-you/nutrition/calculate-my-calcium).

In the table on the following page is a list of foods that you may want to consider integrating more of into your regular diet. Included there are the approximate amounts of calcium in each of these foods. If you wish to consume little or no milk products and want other options for foods rich in calcium, try drinking fortified beverages (i.e., brands with added calcium), or eating calcium rich vegetables and legumes (e.g., beans, spinach, broccoli). Appropriate portions of these foods (e.g., a cup of cooked broccoli or beans as a side dish) may not be as rich a source of calcium, but do offer some variety to your diet.

For more information on calcium content in foods, visit the website of the Office of Dietary Supplements (National Institutes of Health, ods.od.nih.gov), or you can look up the nutrient information of any food by visiting the U.S. Department of Agriculture website (ndb.nal.usda.gov).

| Source of Calcium | Serving Size | Approximate Amount of Calcium (mg) |
| --- | --- | --- |
| Yogurt (plain, low-fat) | 1 cup | 415 |
| Canned sardines (in oil, including bones) | 85 g (3 oz) | 325 |
| Cheddar cheese | 43 g (1.5 oz) | 310 |
| Milk (whole, skim, or low-fat) | 1 cup | 300 |
| Soy Milk (calcium-fortified) | 1 cup | 300 |
| Orange juice (calcium-fortified) | 3/4 cup | 260 |
| Tofu (firm, made with calcium sulfate) | 1/2 cup | 250 |
| Canned salmon (pink, including bones) | 85 g (3 oz) | 180 |
| Cottage cheese (1% milk fat) | 1 cup | 140 |
| Kale (raw) | 1 cup | 100 |
| Frozen yogurt (vanilla, soft serve) | 1/2 cup | 100 |
| Sesame seeds (whole, dried) | 1 tbsp. | 88 |
| Broccoli (raw) | 1 cup | 42 |
| Chick-peas (canned) | 1/2 cup | 38 |
| Bread (whole-wheat) | 1 slice | 30 |
| Sweet potato (baked) | 1/2 cup | 30 |
| Cream cheese (regular) | 1 tbsp. | 14 |

**RECOMMENDATION:**

Calcium intake of up to 1,000–1,200 mg daily, preferably from diet (with 600–800 IU of vitamin D), is recommended for general health and to prevent bone loss and fractures.

## Phytonutrients

Phytonutrients ("phyto" = plant) refer to a wide range of compounds in plant foods that promote health and are associated with a lower risk of cancer. Phytonutrients are different from vitamins and minerals found in plant foods and also have health benefits.

### Polyphenols

Polyphenols are antioxidants found in many fruits and vegetables and are known to reduce the risk of getting cancer, at least in animal studies. Antioxidants protect your cells from damage that can lead to disease. The isoflavones found in soy are an example of compounds with strong antioxidant properties. Cruciferous vegetables, such as broccoli, cauliflower, cabbage, and kale, are high in antioxidants, but they are found in many other foods. Before covering a few more, there is one fact that sometimes gets missed in discussions of phytonutrients and cancer. Although foods rich in antioxidants can lower the risk of getting cancer, there is no convincing evidence that a diet rich in vegetables or even a vegan diet alone will cure prostate cancer.

No foods rich in phytonutrients are known to cure prostate cancer, and there are no foods or supplements known to be more beneficial than an overall well-balanced diet.

### Punicalagin and Ellagic Acid

Pomegranate is a rich source of polyphenols including the antioxidant punicalagin. A second type of polyphenol, ellagic acid, can be found in the red berrylike seeds inside the fruit. Interest in pomegranates' antioxidant effects, along with promising early research with animals and in test tubes, has encouraged the study of pure pomegranate juice in men treated for prostate cancer. Although the research is promising, it is too soon to draw conclusions about the benefit of pomegranates or their juice for men on ADT. Because of its increased popularity, pomegranate juice can now be found in the produce section of most grocery stores. Pomegranate juice is high in sugar, though so limit your intake to one to two cups a day.

### Lycopene

Lycopene is a type of polyphenol antioxidant found primarily in tomatoes (it is what makes them red), as well as in papaya and watermelon. Although research into the links between lycopene and prostate cancer prevention is promising, not all studies have found a relationship between them. Tomatoes and other fruits also contain a wide range of other nutrients important to health and are recommended as part of a diet rich in plant-based foods. We do know that lycopene from natural sources is widely available, safe to eat, and can easily be incorporated into your diet.

Fresh fruits and vegetables aren't necessarily the best way to get lycopene. Cooked tomatoes (in sauces and juices) are better than fresh ones because lycopene is fat-soluble: Your body will absorb more lycopene when it is processed with a little oil. Cooking tomatoes is also preferred, since heat releases lycopene from inside the plant cells. It is best to select low-salt, low-sugar versions of tomato juice, sauce, and paste.

The following table will help you determine the lycopene concentration in common foods:

| Food | Measure | Lycopene Content (mg) |
| --- | --- | --- |
| Vegetable juice cocktail | 1 cup | 23 |
| Tomato juice | 1 cup | 22 |
| Pasta sauce | 1/2 cup | 22 |
| Watermelon | 1 wedge (about 286 g) | 13 |
| Tomato soup (canned, made with milk) | 1 cup | 13 |
| Stewed tomatoes | 1 cup | 10 |
| Raw tomato | 1 tomato (about 123 g) | 3 |
| Ketchup | 1 tbsp | 3 |
| Grapefruit | 1/2 grapefruit (about 123 g) | 2 |

Making lifestyle changes in order to eat better, like those suggested in this chapter, can be challenging. You may have trouble convincing yourself that it is worthwhile. This is a good opportunity to use a Pros/Cons table to convince yourself that for all the effort, the benefits will outweigh the inconvenience! Involve your partner and/or your other loved ones to support you in your decision, and maybe they will make the change to eating healthy with you. Know that it gets easier with time, as your new lifestyle becomes a habit.

## Activity: Pros/Cons Table

Managing the side effects of ADT often requires making substantial changes to your lifestyle. Sometimes, even though you *want* to make a lifestyle change, you may need to persuade yourself that the change is in fact worthwhile. The Pros/Cons table can be helpful in evaluating a decision to change your eating habits. Here's an example of such a table:

Now, try it out for yourself.

|  | PROS | CONS |
|---|---|---|
| **MAKING THE CHANGE:** <br> Eating at home more | • better for my health <br> • save money <br> • spend more time with my partner cooking in the kitchen <br> • learn a new skill <br> • feel better about the healthy decision I've made | • requires effort <br> • requires more planning <br> • takes time |
| **STAYING THE SAME:** <br> Continuing to eat out routinely | • easier; requires less effort <br> • get to keep eating foods I enjoy | • I will probably gain weight <br> • feel disappointed in myself for not changing |

|  | PROS | CONS |
|---|---|---|
| **MAKING THE CHANGE:** |  |  |
| **STAYING THE SAME:** |  |  |

## Activity: Action Plan · · · · · · · · · · · · · · · · · · · · · · ·

The concept of action plans was introduced in more detail in Chapter 2 on p. 21. Here is an example of how you might complete an Action Plan to make healthy eating choices.

### Action Plan Example: Reduce Eating Out

**What I plan to do**: plan my meals ahead so I don't resort to eating out when I'm too tired or don't have any ideas about what to make

**When I plan to do it**: Saturday—develop a meal plan, grocery list, and go shopping

**Who I might do it with**: my partner

**Why my plan is important**: so I feel better about myself, have better health and improved energy levels, and save money

**Where I plan to do it**: in my home

**What might get in the way?** inconvenience

**How I will address what might get in the way**: planning ahead will help me to prepare food ahead of time so that healthy options are ready and accessible rather than falling back on eating out

## Activity: Goal Setting and Confidence · · · · · · · · · · · · · · ·

First, identify which of your goals you are rating. In order to support your goal, it is helpful to ask yourself how confident you are that you can be successful in making this change.

Write down your goal.

**Goal:** _____

(e.g., reduce frequency of eating out)

i) Rate how confident you feel that you'll achieve your nutrition goal:

| 1 | 2 | 3 | 4 | 5 | 6 | 7 | 8 | 9 | 10 |
|---|---|---|---|---|---|---|---|---|---|

Not confident                                                    Very confident

ii) Rate how motivated you are to accomplish your nutrition goal:

| 1 | 2 | 3 | 4 | 5 | 6 | 7 | 8 | 9 | 10 |
|---|---|---|---|---|---|---|---|---|---|

Not motivated                                                   Very motivated

iii) Rate how likely you are to actually carry out your nutrition goal:

| 1 | 2 | 3 | 4 | 5 | 6 | 7 | 8 | 9 | 10 |
|---|---|---|---|---|---|---|---|---|---|

Not likely                                                        Very likely

## Healthy Eating: Essentials

ADT has several side effects that can be reduced with a well-balanced diet and a healthy lifestyle. In addition to side effects, such as loss of muscle mass and weight gained as fat, men on ADT are also at increased risk of osteoporosis, diabetes, and cardiovascular problems. In this chapter, we outlined how eating healthy can help you manage your weight and reduce these risk factors.

In general, you should aim for the following:
1. Eat less saturated and trans fats.
2. Eat more high-fiber foods.
3. Limit salt and sugar intake.
4. Eat more fish and less red meat.
5. Eat less processed and junk foods.

In addition, we discuss fats, proteins, and carbohydrates, as well as outline a diet for men being treated with ADT; that is, a diet composed of 20% to 35% fat (no more than 10% from saturated sources), 10% to 35% protein, and 45% to 65% carbohydrates. Add foods rich in phytonutrients, such as soy and tomatoes to your diet. Also include 600 to 800 IU of vitamin D per day alongside no more than 1,200 mg calcium per day from all sources. These are important components of a healthy diet for men on ADT, in particular for bone health.

## Moving Forward: Questions for Discussion

- What has been my daily caloric intake for the past three days?
- Did I get any soy in my diet? If so how many different forms of soy have I eaten in the last week? If I have not been eating soy, what is one way that I could introduce it into my diet this coming week?
- What actions have I taken (or can I take) to cut back on the amount of saturated fats that I have eaten in the past three days?
- What are some foods that I can eat to introduce more natural sources of calcium into my diet?
- How many servings of fish have I eaten in the last week?
- Are there opportunities for me to reduce my salt or sugar intake?
- What are some ways I can become more involved in grocery shopping and meal planning so as to rely less on prepared/convenience food items and eating out?
- What are some of the lasting mental health benefits that I might begin to notice if I start eating better?

**NOTES:**

_____

_____

_____

_____

_____

_____

_____

_____

_____

_____

_____

_____

_____

_____

_____

_____

_____

# 5

# Effects on Psychological Well-Being

A diagnosis of cancer and subsequent adjustment to the effects of cancer treatment often leaves patients and loved ones feeling stressed, which can come to the surface as changes in emotions and mood. Both patients and partners report changes in emotions after men start undergoing ADT, such as mood swings or increased emotional expression, often referred to as *emotional lability*. It is perfectly normal for you to experience abrupt mood changes, depression, anxiety, and grief during ADT treatment. It is important for you to be aware of this and to be open to discussion about changes in emotional responses or sensitivity that might occur.

Emotional lability can create challenges for relationships. If the patient thinks that his new and heightened emotions are wrong and must be hidden or denied, his desire to draw on social support from others can be compromised. Patients may also experience depression, anxiety, and grief that can be difficult to adjust to.

Emotional changes can be quite variable. Some men may become angry, bitter, and/or pessimistic while on ADT. Others may become more sentimental and openly tearful. Often, partners or close friends see the changes before the patient himself notices.

ADT may also impact a patient's **cognitive function**, which refers to conscious thinking processes such as attention, concentration, and memory. The research examining the nature of these changes during ADT is inconsistent.

It is hard to know if changes in cognitive function are natural responses to aging or are brought on by stress, anxiety, depression, and/or fatigue. We believe that you should be aware that ADT *might* affect cognitive function, though we do not know how common such changes in cognitive function are with ADT. If you do notice cognitive changes, such as memory loss, it is also unknown how long those changes may last.

## Emotional Distress

When your PSA rises after completion of primary treatments, such as prostatectomy or radiotherapy, having to start or resume ADT can be associated with significant distress for both you and your loved ones. At this point, we know that the previous, potentially curative, treatments are no longer an option. Some despair is understandable in this situation. These feelings should be balanced against the reality that ADT can help control your cancer for many years, if not decades, to come.

A common stressor for prostate cancer patients centers on having blood drawn for a PSA test and then needing to wait for the results. Patients on ADT are required to have regular PSA tests, and that alone can contribute significantly to the emotional burden of being on ADT.

You are also likely to experience additional stress at various points in the course of your treatment. These reactions are realistic in response to a difficult situation. However, if you find that you are significantly distressed, you should consider additional treatment for depression and/or anxiety.

We can't tell you how you will react to emotional changes that may come with ADT, but we can say that your willingness to talk about such changes can help bring you closer to your loved ones. Others will appreciate you sharing your feelings with them.

At the other extreme, if you feel that you need to deny or hide such changes from your loved ones, it could make things confusing and frustrating for both you and them. Partners often report that patient withdrawal is the hardest thing for them to deal with.

## Emotional Expression

Spontaneous tearfulness is commonly reported by ADT patients; perhaps because it is a noticeable sign of emotional change. In mainstream culture, men or women may feel that it is "unmanly" for a man to shed tears. In reality, there are various reasons why anyone might cry (e.g., physical discomfort, sadness, joy). If you as a patient start to find yourself crying about something that you might never have cried about before, it can be helpful to determine what caused that moment of tearfulness.

One patient on ADT told us that he never teared up because of pain or self-pity; rather, he became tearful in response to news stories and TV advertisements that focused on the triumphs and tribulations of humankind. This patient interpreted his occasional spontaneous tearfulness as a demonstration of heightened empathy for others, and subsequently took personal pride in his newly acquired sensitivity. He now shares tissues with his partner during sentimental movies, and they both feel closer because of his new ability to both show and share emotional responsiveness.

Another patient saw any tendency for tearfulness as a sign of lost masculine strength. He became embarrassed when his family saw him cry, and then got angry with himself for being emotional. He withdrew from his family and would not talk about what happened or how he felt, which pained those who cared about him.

A third patient reported increased expression of anger. This patient told us that he had always been calm and slow to respond when angry. Now he acknowledged that he was shouting and slamming doors. His family had a difficult time figuring out what had happened. Such changes can be confusing for patients, partners, family members, and close friends who have not anticipated the emotional lability that ADT can bring on.

## Activity: Self-Assessment—Screening for Emotional Distress

Many patients and their loved ones experience significant emotional distress when dealing with cancer treatment and ADT. If you are interested in doing a self-assessment, the following questionnaires will give you an idea of how you are doing. Regardless of whether or not you or your loved ones choose to fill out these questionnaires, you may still find it valuable to continue reading the rest of the chapter.

The following questionnaire (The Patient Health Questionnaire (PHQ-9)) is designed to assess different aspects of your mood. Indicate your response using the categories on the right and circle the number that best represents your experience.

**How often have you experienced the following problems in the past two weeks?**

|  | Not at All | Several Days | More Than Half the Days | Nearly Every Day |
|---|---|---|---|---|
| 1. Little interest or pleasure in doing things | 0 | 1 | 2 | 3 |
| 2. Feeling down, depressed, or hopeless | 0 | 1 | 2 | 3 |
| 3. Trouble falling asleep or staying asleep, or sleeping too much | 0 | 1 | 2 | 3 |
| 4. Feeling tired or having little energy | 0 | 1 | 2 | 3 |

(continued)

**How often have you experienced the following problems in the past two weeks?** (*continued*)

| | Not at All | Several Days | More Than Half the Days | Nearly Every Day |
|---|---|---|---|---|
| 5. Poor appetite or overeating | 0 | 1 | 2 | 3 |
| 6. Feeling bad about yourself, or that you are a failure, or that you have let yourself or your family down | 0 | 1 | 2 | 3 |
| 7. Trouble concentrating on things such as reading the newspaper or watching television | 0 | 1 | 2 | 3 |
| 8. Moving or speaking so slowly that other people could have noticed. Or the opposite—being so fidgety or restless that you have been moving around a lot more than usual | 0 | 1 | 2 | 3 |
| 9. Thoughts that you would be better off dead or of hurting yourself in some way | 0 | 1 | 2 | 3 |
| **Column Totals:** | | ____ + | ____ + | ____ |
| **Add Column Totals Together:** | | _____ | | |

*Scoring Instructions:*

- Scores below 5 indicate no concern.
- Scores between 5 and 14 indicate some mild symptoms of difficulty with mood. You may be able to address these by seeking support from family and friends, beginning to work through a self-help book (see the Resources section on p. 135 for suggestions), or making efforts to engage in more rewarding and pleasurable activities in your life.
- Scores of 15 or higher indicate symptoms of depression and likely warrant seeking help from a professional counselor and/or physician.

The following questionnaire (Generalized Anxiety Disorder 7-Item (GAD-7) Scale) is designed to assess symptoms of distress. Using the categories on the right, indicate the most applicable answer for each item.

**How often have you experienced the following problems in the past two weeks?**

| | Not at All | Several Days | More Than Half the Days | Nearly Every Day |
|---|---|---|---|---|
| 1. Feeling nervous, anxious, or on edge | 0 | 1 | 2 | 3 |
| 2. Not being able to stop or control worrying | 0 | 1 | 2 | 3 |

(*continued*)

**How often have you experienced the following problems in the past two weeks?**
(continued)

| | Not at All | Several Days | More Than Half the Days | Nearly Every Day |
|---|---|---|---|---|
| 3. Worrying too much about different things | 0 | 1 | 2 | 3 |
| 4. Trouble relaxing | 0 | 1 | 2 | 3 |
| 5. Being so restless that it's hard to sit still | 0 | 1 | 2 | 3 |
| 6. Becoming easily annoyed or irritable | 0 | 1 | 2 | 3 |
| 7. Feeling afraid, as if something awful might happen | 0 | 1 | 2 | 3 |
| **Column Totals:** | | ____ + | ____ + | ____ |
| **Add Totals Together:** | | _____ | | |

Scoring Instructions:

• Scores below 5 indicate no concern.

• Scores between 5 and 10 indicate some mild symptoms of difficulty with stress. You may be able to address these by seeking support from family and friends, beginning to work through a self-help book (see the Resources section on p. 135 for suggestions), or practicing the relaxation exercises listed below

• Scores over 10 indicate symptoms of anxiety and warrant seeking help from a professional counselor and/or family physician.

## Depression

Although the medical literature varies greatly in its assessment of how common depression is among patients on ADT, patients often report feeling depressed. It is very important to discuss with your physician if you are feeling depressed or have a low mood. There are interventions that can be very helpful, including regular physical activity, psychological counseling, and pharmaceutical treatments.

Depression in cancer patients on ADT rarely appears as a single problem. More often, fatigue, insomnia, and depression form a triad of interrelated symptoms. Because one or more of these complications is frequently a side effect of treatment, it can be difficult to distinguish the primary cause(s) from subsequent effect(s). In fact, it is *not* established that ADT physiologically or directly causes depression. Rather, depression, when it manifests, is more likely an indirect, but entirely realistic, emotional reaction to the situation that ADT patients find themselves in.

It is possible that depression may have little to do with the ADT itself, but rather may be a response to a cancer diagnosis and the many changes that it brings to the lives of all those that it touches. Some studies have suggested that low testosterone from ADT is associated with greater feelings of sadness and low mood, but not all studies have found this. New research also suggests that insulin resistance (diabetes) and a tendency toward depression may be linked. This is another reason why exercise, which helps regulate blood sugar, is so important for the physical and psychological well-being of men on ADT.

Note that rates of depression in the *partners* of cancer patients are often as high as the rates in patients. In fact, one study with prostate cancer couples showed that depression in the partners of patients on ADT was higher than for the patients themselves. Therefore, it *is* important for partners to seek treatment as well, if they feel depressed!

Overall, both patients and partners should be concerned about changes in vitality and spirit. Watch for any of these signs of depression in yourself. You can also watch for these changes in your loved ones:

- Feeling too tired and gloomy to exercise.
- Feeling sadness that doesn't seem to dissipate.
- Becoming withdrawn and noncommunicative.
- Losing interest in a range of personal activities that were previously enjoyable.
- Feeling worthless, guilty, hopeless.
- Having diminished ability to concentrate or make decisions.

## Anxiety

Depression and anxiety often coexist, and may be expressed in similar ways. This can make it particularly hard to decipher the causes for a change in mood. Be aware of the increase in stress in your life associated with the transition to ADT, and remain determined to find time to rest and relax. Some of the best treatments for anxiety and depression include: eating healthy, exercising, having someone to talk to, medication, and/or counseling. Watch for any of these signs of anxiety in yourself and your loved ones:

- Worrying excessively about the future for an extended period of time.
- Fear of "going crazy" or losing control.
- Feeling "on edge" or that you just can't relax.
- Having difficulty sleeping.
- Feeling that your mind is racing.

To live well on ADT, it's important to maintain an active lifestyle and nurture genuine communication with your loved ones. Depression and anxiety can hinder both. The most effective treatment for depression and anxiety involves medication paired with psychotherapy or counseling. Exercise and healthy eating are also effective.

Talk to your doctor, psychologist, or counselor if you are suffering. Timely treatment can set you free to enjoy life again.

## Activity: Progressive Muscle Relaxation ·················

This exercise is to help you learn how to relax your body and mind. Developed by Edmund Jacobsen in the 1920s, *progressive muscle relaxation* is a well-known exercise in which a person tenses and then relaxes the various muscle groups in the body. If you have any pain or discomfort, move on to another muscle group. It may be helpful if, throughout this exercise, you visualize the muscles tensing and then a wave of relaxation flowing over you as you release the tension. Remember to breathe throughout the exercise; don't hold your breath.

Physical tension in the body occurs when we are anxious or stressed. We are often not aware of the tension we hold in our head, jaw, neck, and shoulders until someone brings it to our attention; we do not think to relax these muscle groups. This exercise can be practiced whether you are sitting in a chair or lying down. Make sure to choose a comfortable position. After you have read these instructions, you may choose to practice with your eyes closed if you are comfortable doing so.

You may not want to practice this exercise if you are prone to muscle spasms, or if you have pain from an existing injury.

1. Begin by creating a tight fist with your hands. Hold your arms out straight in front of you and hold this tension. Take note of what the tightness in your muscles feels like. Hold for at least 10 seconds. As you breathe out, relax your fists and let go of any tension you were holding. If you are sitting, allow your arms to fall to your sides and feel the muscles go limp. It is important to deliberately focus on the difference between the tension and relaxation in your muscles. Rest for 20 to 30 seconds.

2. Now move your attention to your feet. Scrunch up your toes into a ball. Then, tense up your ankles, pointing your toes toward your nose. Feel the stretch in the muscles of your calves as you do this. Hold for 10 seconds. Then, while exhaling, release the tension and rest for 20 to 30 seconds.

3. Move your attention up to your thighs and buttocks. Tighten up these muscles so that your body weight is lifted off the surface you are sitting or lying on. Squeeze your thighs together and hold for 10 seconds. Now exhale and feel the release of the tension. Rest for 20 to 30 seconds.

4. Move your attention now to your abdomen. Imagine bringing your belly button closer to your spine and straighten your body. Hold this posture for 10 seconds. Then exhale, releasing the muscle tension and letting all the muscles of your belly (body wall) become loose; feel the tension disappear. Rest here for 20 to 30 seconds.

5. Next, move to your shoulders. Scrunch them up as close to your ears as you can and squeeze your upper arms against your ribcage. Hold for 10 seconds. Exhale, releasing the tension and letting your arms relax away from your body. If you are sitting, your shoulders fall. Rest for 20 to 30 seconds.

6. Now squeeze the muscles in your face. Scrunch up your forehead, eyebrows, eyes, and lips. Close your mouth and gently bite down. Hold for 10 seconds. As you exhale, release the tension and relax for 20 to 30 seconds.

Take a quick mental scan of your body, noting any areas where you are still holding or feeling any tension. Often, as we adjust to relax one area of our body, we begin to tense another area without being aware that we are doing so. Repeat any of the steps above to ensure that you have let go of all of the tension in that muscle group. Try to perform this progressive muscle relaxation once or twice daily.

Like other things in life, practicing this exercise will improve your skill over time. When you begin, it may take you 20 minutes to complete the exercise and even then you may not become fully relaxed. With consistent practice, though, you will find that it takes you only a few minutes to fully relax. An alternative relaxation exercise is the abdominal breathing technique detailed on pages 12 to 13 as a treatment for hot flashes. Introducing relaxation exercises or deep breathing into your daily routine may help you to manage overall chronic stress or anxiety.

## Fatigue

You should not confuse the bodily feeling of muscle fatigue that you get at the end of a strenuous exercise session with the mental fatigue that comes from not exercising. Pushing your body by exercising increases blood flow to the muscles you are working, as well as to the brain. Right after exercising in this way, your body may feel tired, but you will sleep better and your brain will feel more alert in the following days.

## Grief

Cancer and cancer treatments bring with them many changes, including changes interpreted as losses. With ADT, changes that affect how a man feels in terms of his vitality and sexuality may surface. For some men these changes are minor, but for many they are very significant. For many men it may be difficult to accept transitions or losses brought on by ADT that affect their core identity and sense of self. It is okay to grieve losses. In fact, much has been written in the cancer literature about how important grieving is to the process of recovering from loss. Grieving is therapeutic.

Among the changes associated with ADT there are those linked with a man's body image, as well as a man's

Grieving losses from ADT can be difficult because the changes may be more internal and emotional, and hard to articulate to others or even to oneself. Patients on ADT typically know they have changed, but for many it is not easy to describe exactly how they are experiencing those changes.

sense of physical strength and masculinity. ADT can change how a man's body feels, and how he feels about his body. These changes can negatively impact a patient's mood, attitude, and thoughts; how a man thinks and feels about both himself and his partner. How easily you, either as a patient or as a loved one, adapt to these changes can be influenced by how willing you are to acknowledge and accept the changes in the first place.

After the effects of ADT take shape, you may find it helpful to make a list of the things you consider lost or reduced due to ADT. Some examples may be physical strength, loss of spontaneous sex, decreased erectile function, loss of libido, and changes to your body form and physical appearance.

> People grieve in different ways—some may cry about a specific loss, while others may choose a designated time to remember and celebrate the ways things were. Other individuals may reframe loss so they see it as a benefit. Discuss what each loss or change means to both you and to your partner. Then you can make the decision to move ahead with life together, despite those changes.

One of the obstacles to living comfortably with change is an all-too-common effort to try to reestablish or reaffirm life as it was before ADT. Too often this requires pretending that life has not changed. On the surface this may work for the patient, but for partners and loved ones a patient's silence and reluctance to acknowledge change can make the grieving process all that more difficult.

Men often engage in a code of silence. Because men rarely talk with others about aspects of their lives that make them feel less manly, men on ADT may feel culturally trapped into pretending that their lives have not changed. The more that men are reluctant to reveal how they feel after going on ADT, the more other patients assume that being silent is the right thing—the "manly" thing—to do. This leads to a vicious cycle, where masculine culture can make it particularly difficult for patients to acknowledge change and loss during ADT. This traps men into denying change and hiding how they really feel.

The more that patients use denial to deal with the changes that ADT brings to their lives, the less they can grieve. This makes it that much more difficult for them to adapt to the changes they are experiencing and to recover from their losses.

Adapting well to ADT often involves sharing your grief with someone. If you have a partner, it means that both of you are willing to share with and support each other in whatever grief you each may experience along the way. Although this can be painful emotionally, the end-product is often a couple that is closer and more supportive of each other than ever before.

If you share your concerns with a loved one, you may find that your relationships are stronger, not weaker, after ADT. This may allow you to better accept the changes and losses you experience as a result of ADT.

Grief is interlinked with emotional expression. If men feel that it is unmanly to display emotion, yet inside they feel a loss, they may hold their grief inside. Typically, partners know that the patients are troubled by the changes in their lives brought on by their cancer treatment. But if the patients themselves are reluctant to talk about how they are experiencing these changes, partners may feel that the best they can do is to join their men in pretending that little has changed. Ultimately, in this situation, the couple moves farther apart rather than closer together. It is at times like this when couples counseling can be beneficial.

## Cognition

Decreases in testosterone levels in nonprostate cancer patients have been linked to changes in spatial or visual processing, as well as to changes in navigation styles. It is possible, if changes in cognition occur while on ADT, they will be seen in these same areas. In everyday life, such changes can manifest themselves as problems such as not remembering where you left your car keys, or why you went to the fridge in the first place. The ability to remember new words may also be influenced by ADT. However, other research suggests that cognitive impairment with ADT does not occur at all. Rather, these changes, when observed, can be attributed to aging, stress, and illness in general.

Bill Cosby once said that his memory must be in his butt because he would stand up to get something, walk to the room to get the item, forget what he was looking for, and only remember when he sat back down again.

Despite the fact that the cognitive effects of ADT are not well defined, there are ways you can improve or maintain cognitive function, should you experience such problems. The following suggestions are largely preventative and should be started as early as possible, before cognitive changes affect one's daily life.

- *Maintain an active lifestyle.* Exercising improves blood flow throughout your body, including the brain. Improving blood flow helps your brain to work faster, improving cognitive abilities such as memory, attention, and concentration.
- *Keep your brain active.* Do activities that make your brain work, including reading and conversing with others. Puzzles and games (e.g., sudoku, crossword puzzles, bridge, scrabble) can help you maintain spatial and verbal skills. A variety of games that challenge different parts of your brain (e.g., mathematical ability, memory, logic puzzles, word games) may be best.
- *Be practical.* For example, it helps to have a standard place to keep your car keys. Keep a notebook and pen or pencil by the telephone to write down messages. Get rid of clutter on your desk to help you find things more easily.
- *Focus by avoiding multitasking.* If you have something important to write or to read (like this book!), give it your full attention without TV, radio, or other distracting noises in the background.

- *Write important things down.* For example, write your appointments on a calendar that you keep clearly visible, or write them down in an agenda.
- *Medications.* There are medications that are being developed to help slow the mental decline that we all experience with aging. So far, one small, short-term study has suggested that estradiol can help slow memory decline from ADT.

### Activity: Pros/Cons Table . . . . . . . . . . . . . . . . . . .

If you have been reading through this book chapter by chapter, you are familiar with the value of the Pros/Cons exercise by now. This exercise can be applied to any decision in your life. Below is an example of the Pros/Cons exercise related to addressing emotional concerns.

|  | PROS | CONS |
|---|---|---|
| **MAKING THE CHANGE:**<br>Seeing a counselor | • They might have ideas about how to help with my stress<br>• They might be able to assure me that I am doing just fine and then I don't have to worry<br>• They might be able to provide additional support for my partner<br>• My partner might be relieved that I am getting support | • It could be embarrassing to ask for help<br>• Have to take time out of my schedule for appointments<br>• There may be an additional cost |
| **DON'T CHANGE:**<br>Continue without seeing a counselor | • I don't have to face the reality that maybe I need some extra support<br>• I don't have to feel embarrassed | • I might continue to struggle<br>• I feel overwhelmed and unsupported<br>• My partner feels overwhelmed trying to support me |

Now, try it out for yourself.

|  | PROS | CONS |
|---|---|---|
| **MAKING THE CHANGE:** |  |  |
| **STAYING THE SAME:** |  |  |

## Activity: Action Plan

Again you are reminded that it is best to start small with something very manageable (e.g., walking regularly) before you take on larger scale goals (e.g., running a 10-km race). Post your completed form somewhere where you will see it every day, like next to your bathroom mirror, to remind yourself of your commitment to this goal.

### Action Plan Example: Work on Stress Management

**What I plan to do:** use the progressive muscle relaxation exercise regularly

**When I plan to do it:** every day at lunch break for 15 minutes

**Who I might do it with:** by myself

**Why my plan is important:** to improve my ability to manage chronic stress and to build my relaxation skills

**Where I plan to do it:** at my desk, with the door closed, after I have eaten my lunch

**What might get in the way?** people might think I am weird, or wonder what I am doing

**How I will address what might get in the way:** I will close my office door

Here is a blank copy that you can fill out. An additional copy is located in the Appendix on page 124. It helps to be as specific as possible when you are making your Action Plan.

**Action Plan:** _____

What I plan to do: _____

_____

When I plan to do it: _____

_____

Who I might do it with: _____

_____

Why my plan is important: _____

_____

Where I plan to do it: _____

_____

What might get in the way? _____

_____

How I will address what might get in the way: _____

_____

## Activity: Goal Setting and Confidence · · · · · · · · · · · · · · · ·

In order to support your goal, take a moment to rate the following factors associated with your goal. First, write down your goal (this might be what you have written in your Action Plan):

**Goal:** _____

i) Rate how confident you feel that you'll achieve your goal:

| 1 | 2 | 3 | 4 | 5 | 6 | 7 | 8 | 9 | 10 |
|---|---|---|---|---|---|---|---|---|----|

Not confident　　　　　　　　　　　　　　　　Very confident

ii) Rate how motivated you are to accomplish your goal:

| 1 | 2 | 3 | 4 | 5 | 6 | 7 | 8 | 9 | 10 |
|---|---|---|---|---|---|---|---|---|----|

Not motivated　　　　　　　　　　　　　　　　Very motivated

iii) Rate how likely you are to actually carry out your goal:

| 1 | 2 | 3 | 4 | 5 | 6 | 7 | 8 | 9 | 10 |
|---|---|---|---|---|---|---|---|---|----|

Not likely　　　　　　　　　　　　　　　　　　Very likely

If any of your answers *are less than 5*:

- Consider either enlisting the help of a friend to hold you accountable or implementing a reward system to help motivate you (see pages 42–43 for additional information on motivation, lapses, relapses, rewards, and support).
- Consider revising your goal—Is it too ambitious a goal to start with? Can you start with a more modest goal and work your way up to a more significant lifestyle change?
- Remind yourself—What are the reasons? Why you want to make this change? What potential benefits may you notice? List these on a piece of paper and refer back to them when you are feeling particularly unmotivated.
- Consider completing the previous Pros/Cons table to help you identify your motivations (pros) for making this change, but also some of the barriers (cons) that might be getting in the way of making the change.

## Effects on Psychological Well-Being: Essentials

Some patients report that they experience no changes in their mood, emotions, or thought process while undergoing ADT. Others notice significant changes that make them uncomfortable. We encourage you to be aware of the possibility of change, and should changes occur, take simple steps to address and accommodate them.

Some of the psychological changes that can occur with ADT, such as depression or anxiety, can be helped by exercise, medication, and counseling. If changes in memory occur, they can often be compensated for by small changes in lifestyle and working habits. Planning can be a very important factor in adapting successfully to change. Remember to talk to your health care team if these problems arise so that they can be addressed properly.

Emotional changes (particularly increased tearfulness), although common, are not necessarily negative. They can even be seen as enriching your life if you accept them as positive signs of your sensitivity to others, and not as a loss of masculine detachment and reserve.

Changes in mood, emotions, or cognition are often very subtle and may be noticed by a partner or loved one before they are noticed or acknowledged by a patient. Not talking about these changes when they are obvious to others can hurt relationships. They are not uniformly bad, and they do not need to be hidden. Talking about any changes is very important for adapting to them.

## Moving Forward: Questions for Discussion

### Emotional Changes:

- How will I acknowledge and communicate with my loved ones about any changes in my mood and emotions that I experience on ADT?
- How do I feel about increased emotional expression?
- What will I do if I become depressed or experience anxiety?
- What will I do if my loved ones become depressed or experience anxiety?
- What things have I lost since having cancer and starting ADT?
- What can I do to help grieve something that I have lost?

### Cognitive Changes:

- How do I feel about cognitive changes, for example, increased forgetfulness?
- What can I incorporate into my life to prevent or reduce the impact of cognitive changes?
- What changes can I make around the house or office to help me if cognitive changes occur?
- How will I explain this effect of ADT to my friends and family if they notice a change?

**NOTES:**

# 6

# Effects on Intimate Relationships and Sexuality

This chapter is relevant to couples who stopped having intercourse before ADT as well as those who were sexually active before starting ADT. We have found that a loss of libido changes most couples' relationships—even those who were not previously sexually active.

Even if you are single, you may find this section relevant as you may find yourself in a relationship in the future. Also, even outside of a relationship you are a sexual being, and will likely notice many of these changes.

## ADT Lowers Libido

Approximately 90% of men on ADT experience a reduction of libido (desire for sex). A reduction in libido typically leads to a reduction in the frequency of sexual activity, and in some cases a complete cessation of sexual activity. Reductions in libido can also lead

> One partner shared with us: "I was very afraid of living together like brother and sister. It feels like you're going to move into this platonic sort of relationship where there's none of that wonderful thing you had as a husband and wife."

to fewer displays of physical affection. ADT may thus bring special challenges to relationships. A reduced libido has implications to not just the patient on ADT but also to his intimate partner.

### How the Loss of Libido Affects Couples

Couples respond to the loss of libido from ADT in many different ways:

- Some couples may not have been having sex at the time of treatment and may notice little change.
- Some couples readily accept the loss of sex in exchange for a potentially longer life.
- Some couples may stop having sex and find that they experience sorrow and mourn the loss of their sex life.
- With the loss of sexual intimacy, some couples stop being physically affectionate and this can contribute to a sense of disconnection between partners.
- Some couples redefine their sexual activity and focus on those activities that they are still able to do, finding new joy in that.

As a patient on ADT, you may feel that you have lost your zest for life. You may no longer find delight in flirting because it does not feel genuine. You may long for the thrill of getting lost in a sexual fantasy or simply admiring an attractive person. Your partner may feel grief over the loss of the glances and touches that you used to share. This may lead your partner to feel less appreciated and less desirable. Changes in libido and/or sexual functioning can make it difficult to maintain physical and nonphysical intimacy, both of which are important for maintaining a feeling of closeness.

> One patient said that he likes that he can cuddle up with his wife and enjoy her company without the "carrying on of the last 30 years trying to plan how … to get my wife to have sex."

Here, we explore ways that couples can remain close—or perhaps become even closer—despite the impact of ADT on libido. We present a range of possibilities that require couples to remain open to discussing what a changed libido might mean to them. A prerequisite to maintaining intimacy in the face of reduced libido is successful communication.

### Staying Close in Nonsexual Ways

Intimacy is the feeling of closeness and connection you have with your partner. Intimacy comes from sharing something with someone that you share with no one else. This includes both physical (sexual and nonsexual) and nonphysical contact. While ADT may reduce sexual intimacy, couples can still feel very close and enjoy nonsexual and nonphysical intimacy. For most couples, intimacy is an important part of their relationship, but building intimacy does not necessarily require sex.

Nonphysical intimacy can increase after ADT for many reasons. For example, a cancer diagnosis itself may remind people how precious their relationships are, and a stronger appreciation for each other (one that is not driven solely by sexual desire) can develop or be strengthened. Also, mismatched libido could have been a source of tension in some partnerships prior to ADT. For example, when a man on ADT who previously had a higher sex drive now has a drive that matches his partner, this can ease tension if both partners are accepting of the change.

When ADT reduces a patient's desire for sexual intimacy and his ability to have erections, many couples stop penetrative activities, including sexual intercourse. Refraining from sexual intercourse is common and is not, in itself, problematic if both partners are okay with that. What can lead to problems is when couples in this situation become less physically affectionate overall. This can result in both partners longing for the comfort that physical affection brings, whether through cuddling, hugs, kisses, or even orgasms. At the same time, partners or patients may be holding back because they fear that expressing physical affection may cause anxiety, pressure, or expectations of a sexual nature. For example, the patient may think: "I don't want to be too physically affectionate because I don't want to start something sexual that I can't finish"; his partner may think: "I don't want to cuddle up to him because he'll assume it means I want sexual intercourse and that will just make him feel worse."

> One man told us that without sexual urges reminding him of the importance of showing affection to his wife, he seldom thought of it.
>
> His solution was to wear a prostate cancer bracelet on his wrist. Whenever he felt it, he either made a point of telling his wife something that he appreciated about her or touched her affectionately.

Try discussing what you each consider to be physical affection that leads to sexual intercourse or other sexual activities, compared to physical affection that can simply be interpreted as being close and enjoying each other's warmth. You may decide that holding hands, hugging, cuddling, or kissing are physically intimate activities you can enjoy without either of you feeling obligated to move toward further sexual activity. If you communicate beforehand, and you each know which activities mean closeness without committing to sex, and which activities mean you have an interest in sex, you can reduce anxiety and false expectations. This can help you continue to enjoy each other's company and stay affectionate.

The key is to communicate about your expectations and know that you can be physically affectionate without that affection needing to lead to sexual activity.

You may experience a whole range of emotions when it comes to how your sexuality has been affected by ADT. You may feel anxious about being intimate with your partner, in sexual or nonsexual ways, because your sex drive and ability to perform have been affected. You may be self-conscious about how your body or your genitalia look after long-term treatment. You may be angry that you do not have the sex drive you had before going on ADT, and may feel ashamed or see yourself as less manly because of your reduced sex drive.

If you feel any of these things, it can help to acknowledge your feelings and openly discuss them with your partner. Sharing your concerns can help to build relational intimacy and also help you to cope with negative feelings.

## Making Time for Intimacy

One couple told us about their sexual encounters: "We have positive experiences. I think it maintains a closeness if nothing else. Our sexual relationship is different now, but the fact that we want to give pleasure to each other is good, even if it doesn't happen very often."

One suggestion for adapting sexually to the impact of ADT on intimacy is to choose one evening a week as a "date night." This way, you do not have to rely on your bodies reminding you to share physical intimacy, even if that intimacy is not sexual. It may help you to realize that when we're not hungry for food, looking at the clock reminds us to eat so we do not ignore our nutritional needs. When we're not hungry for sex, looking at the "date night" note on the calendar reminds us to feed each other's need for physical and emotional intimacy, whether sexual or not. If you often feel tired in the evening, consider moving your lovemaking to the morning, when you may feel more refreshed.

Here are just a few ideas about how to "sensualize the setting":

- Put on some favorite music and dance together.
- Take a bubble bath together.
- Massage each other.
- Spend time holding each other.
- Enjoy long kisses.
- Spend time touching each other sensually.

Know that the purpose of these activities is to strengthen your physical connection—activities may not, and need not, lead to more explicit sexual activities.

## Sexuality and You

*Note: This section is for patients and their partners who desire a sexual relationship.*

Some of the suggestions in the following discussion of sexuality may go beyond what you are comfortable with. We include explicit descriptions of sexual practices and activities. You may be surprised to learn that some couples continue to enjoy sex despite undergoing ADT. If you, too, desire to maintain sexual intimacy, you are encouraged to communicate openly with your partner to establish what you both are willing to try or not try. Proceed with an open mind.

Sexuality starts with how you feel about yourself overall. It is not just about your body parts. You may choose to express your sexuality in different ways: by the way you dress, by the way you groom yourself, by the way you carry yourself, by the ways in which you have sex, and whom you choose to have sex with. Sexuality, particularly with couples, usually includes caring for someone else intimately. The role that sexuality plays in your life is affected by many factors, including age, environment, health, culture, beliefs, relationships, opportunities, and interests.

Testosterone is one thing that affects your sex drive and sexual performance, but it is not the only thing. Physical and psychological details, such as anxiety and weight gain, can also significantly affect how you view yourself and consequently how you perform sexually. It is important to consider how you view yourself and your partner, and make an effort to think positively about sex.

The brain has a major influence on sexuality. If you are anxious, worried, or depressed, it will be harder to be turned on by the thought of sex. Sometimes it is easy to forget why sexual activities between you and your partner can be so beneficial. Some of the benefits are:

- Provides an opportunity to be close and connected, both physically and emotionally.
- Increases blood circulation and releases muscle tensions.
- Releases hormones that help you relax.

Some worry that becoming sexually aroused will raise testosterone levels and promote cancer growth. Be assured that this is *NOT* the case.

### Suggestions for Enjoying Sensual Pleasure with Low Libido

Couples undergoing ADT often find that they can no longer rely on spontaneous sexual urges to spark physical intimacy because of the patient's reduced libido. Of course, independent of ADT, as individuals get older, spontaneous desire for sexual interactions usually declines, so changes in levels of desire and interest in sexual intimacy naturally change over the course and length of a relationship.

Although, as a couple, you may have been used to sexual spontaneity before starting ADT, this does not mean you have to give up on all sexuality.

Sexual intimacy may still flourish if the setting is carefully prepared. Part of what makes a meal elegant is the planning that goes into it: opening a bottle of wine, putting on some nice music, and lighting candles. In a similar way, sensuality may be enhanced by planning the time and place for sexual intimacy. It also helps to be open-minded to exploring new things that you may not have done before, but be sure to plan together and communicate your ideas and expectations.

### Be Flexible about Who Initiates Intimacy

One of the most important factors for maintaining physical intimacy after ADT is being flexible about who initiates sexual intimacy. If the partner now has stronger sexual urges than the patient, he or she may need to take the lead in initiating physical affection. For a partner, being the initiator of physical intimacy may be a new and different experience. If the patient has typically been the initiator, being pursued may be new for him. For this shift in roles to work well for both individuals, both partners need to be clear on expectations which means that you have to have talked about your expectations with each other, ahead of time. Discussing the feelings associated with asking one another to engage in physically intimate activities can help prevent misconceptions. Sometimes, initially, it helps to remove the expectation that initiating pleasurable sensual activities must lead to intercourse and orgasm. Removing this expectation helps to decrease any anxiety associated with the feeling that either of you has to "perform" as you did before ADT. Accepting such changes in the roles of who initiates sensual play can work for both partners—if they both communicate about expectations.

### Redefine Your Sexual Activities

Often, when people think of *sex*, they think specifically of penetrative intercourse. At the same time, many people (notably most women) also recognize that there can be much pleasure and sensuality in other forms of sexual interaction. It may represent a change from your focus before ADT, but try to approach sexuality with a focus on pleasure in a broad sense. Foreplay (i.e., the physical activity leading up to sexual intercourse) is an important part of sex and can be enjoyed even in the absence of intercourse (or orgasm) because of the closeness and attention your partner gives to you during this activity. Women generally have lower libidos than men, yet can still enjoy both sexual intercourse and nonpenetrative sexual activities. Men can, too. Experiencing enjoyable sexual activity on ADT requires an understanding that all encounters of pleasure and sensuality do *not* need to end with intercourse or orgasm. Each partner needs to understand how things have changed and be willing to give more attention to sensual touching, caressing, cuddling, and other aspects of sexual play. You may find that with a fresh approach to pleasure and sensuality you and your partner discover (or rediscover) ways of being intimate that meet each other's needs for physical affection.

> With open discussion and conscious attention, activities focusing on pleasure and sensuality can be highly rewarding, and can build intimacy in ways that have been forgotten or have not been used before.

### Take the Focus Off Orgasm

Commonly, in heterosexual couples, for a male with strong sexual urges the ultimate goal of a sexual encounter is orgasm, but with a reduced libido, it becomes more difficult for a man to achieve orgasms. This can become a problem for a man who stops making physical contact with his partner because he doesn't want to start anything he isn't motivated to, or doesn't feel capable of finishing. However, as mentioned earlier, it is essential for the person on ADT to realize that physical contact that does not lead to orgasm is still vitally important for both him and his partner.

### Be Aware of Decreased Responsiveness to Sexual Touch

ADT and the lack of testosterone are associated with decreased sensitivity to erotic touch. Therefore, as a man on ADT, you may not get the same genital pleasure or skin responses that you once did when your partner touched you. A man in this situation needs to be aware that emotional and physical attention is a sign of his partner's caring. He must be careful not to simply reject this touch because it is not as sexually alluring as it may have been in the past. Sadly, those who ignore a partner's advances may hurt the partner, causing feelings of rejection. This may discourage further attempts to initiate physical intimacy, which can undermine intimacy overall and weaken a couple's bond.

Partners of patients on ADT need to know that lowered sex drive and limited responsiveness to sexual advances are *not rejections of them* as persons, partners, or lovers. Patients should be aware, however, that muted responses from them might be interpreted that way. Open discussion can help avoid the risk of the partner misconstruing a patient's low response to sexual stimulation as general rejection.

As an exercise in communication, and to rekindle sensual experiences with your partner, try the mindfulness exercise on pages 99 to 100. Initially, the mindfulness exercise may be practiced on your own. The skill that is built by practicing mindfulness is in attending to all elements of your experience. Turning your attention toward sensations of touch, sight, sound, and so on. Rather than getting distracted by thoughts, judgments, or feelings about a sexual experience (or even about other topics entirely), you can train yourself to bring your attention back to the physical sensations you are experiencing. This type of exercise also helps to foster an appreciation for new experiences or types of sexual stimulation. Practicing mindful awareness during sexual or sensual activity can help to promote increased awareness and enjoyment of physical sensations. Once you have tried the mindfulness exercise on your own a few times, you may wish to use this approach when engaging sexually with your partner.

### Stimulate Your Sexual Appetite

The French axiom, *"L'appetit vient en mangeant,"* or *"Appetite comes while we eat,"* captures the concept of pleasure and sensuality without pressure for intercourse. It resonates with the experience of many couples, especially for those on ADT. Most of us have experienced a lack of an appetite for food; the mere idea of being expected to eat an entire four-course meal when we are not particularly hungry mutes our willingness to take the first bite. However, if we are gently invited to take a taste knowing that we can just nibble the bits that we find appealing and stop when we are full, we can often enjoy the food, and may even find that our appetite is stronger than we thought. Similarly, many men on ADT are more willing to engage in sensual touching when there is no pressure to reach climax or to engage in activities that don't seem appealing. To stay with the food metaphor, one can have a grand meal made up of only the most elegant appetizers without eating a main course. It is possible for a male with both erectile dysfunction and low libido to learn to enjoy sensuality, and sexual pleasure, without reaching an orgasm.

> L'appetit vient en mangeant
> Appetite comes while we eat

One way to stimulate the sexual appetite is to use erotic material. Erotic material comes in many forms: movies, books, short stories, poetry, music, magazines, works of art, and even educational programs. Erotic material often provides a good starting point to increase one's arousal or awareness of physical touch. Bear in mind that erotic material does not necessarily mean pornographic material. Pornography typically focuses on the visual representation of explicit sexual acts, while

> One woman said "I bought some sexy underwear and ... I just laid a path [of rose petals] through to the bedroom. It obviously didn't change his libido but it led to a lot of laughter and that seems to have been a huge missing factor."

erotica is usually subtler and tends to imply sexual interest rather than explicitly show sex organs. Erotic material may or may not arouse a patient with a low libido, but even if it does not help him with arousal, watching or reading erotic material together may serve to draw partners closer together, and open them up to exploring new options.

There is an abundance of erotic material available. We have included some websites and books in the Resources (p. 135) section to get you started. If you browse through them and find something that you are uncomfortable with, or that does not fit your taste, then skip it and select another. You may not know what you or your partner will find interesting or arousing until you try it.

## Orgasms without Ejaculation

If you had other treatments for prostate cancer before ADT, such as a radical prostatectomy or radiotherapy, you may have had an orgasm but with little or no ejaculation. If you haven't had prior treatment for prostate cancer, you are likely to discover that without testosterone you produce little or no seminal fluid when you ejaculate. Thus, even if you had a functioning prostate gland before, it will probably become inactive when you are on ADT.

The absence of ejaculate does not mean that there can be no orgasm, just as the absence of an erection does not mean there can be no orgasm. An orgasm can be thought of as a pelvic sneeze. With sneezes, there is a buildup of tension followed by a release. Or the sneeze can be stifled and the tension can disappear on its own. While a normal sneeze in one's head releases facial tension, an orgasm releases sexual tension. We can have wet sneezes or dry sneezes—they feel different but both are unmistakably sneezes. Similarly, a person can have wet orgasms (with ejaculate) or dry orgasms (with no ejaculate).

Again, these will feel different, but both are orgasms. Some couples celebrate that dry orgasms mean less mess; for some partners, dry orgasms make oral sex more enjoyable.

## Erectile Dysfunction

**Erectile dysfunction (ED)** is increasingly common as men age and is a common side effect of primary prostate cancer treatments (e.g., external beam radiation, prostatectomy). The addition of ADT greatly increases the likelihood of ED. There are ways to restore the capability of having erections. However, the reduced libido of patients on ADT compounds the problem.

Many men on ADT tell us they still enjoy sexual intimacy without erections and with a reduced libido. Sexual activity may look quite different after ADT, but it can still be rewarding for a couple.

Common ED treatments do not work for everyone, and attempting to find the right one can be a frustrating process. Medications used for ED called **phosphodiesterase-5 inhibitors (PDE5i)**—Viagra®, Cialis®, Staxyn®, and Levitra®—are described in detail below. It should be noted that these drugs do not work as well when testosterone levels are low as they do when testosterone levels are in the normal range.

Many men are reluctant to talk to their partners about the use of erectile aids, fearing that they will be seen as inadequate for needing to rely on them, or even more inadequate if the aids don't work for them. Discussing this openly with your partner is important because ED treatments are more effective when the patient's partner is fully informed and even involved in the treatment. Remaining secretive regarding ED treatments may undermine a couple's trust and intimacy in the long run.

## Using Erectile Assistive Aids

While we believe that couples can have mutually satisfying sex without an erection, having an erection and penetrative sex may nevertheless be important for some patients and their partners. Some men find these strategies helpful and effective while others do not. Remember that if the strategy does not work, the failure is in the strategy, not you. It is important to keep an open mind and be willing to try different options, and at times retry some of those that may have failed in the past. If you decide to explore ED treatments there are many options available, ranging from the noninvasive (e.g., PDE5i drugs) to surgical interventions (e.g., penile implants).

With ED treatments you may find that:

- The presence of an erection can help raise your own sexual interest.
- Your partner may become more aroused in the presence of an erection.
- You as a patient can enjoy pleasing your partner, even if you don't have the same quality erection or an orgasm.

But you also may find that:

- The treatment simply does not work; most men on ADT find that common treatments for ED, in particular oral drugs, do not work for them.

It is also possible that erections achieved through ED treatments may be disconcerting in the absence of sexual arousal. However, even if the experience is deemed unsuccessful, your partner may appreciate the effort and time you have taken to explore the options. This can help strengthen your bond as a couple. In other words, exploring new sexual styles and practices together can help maintain and even build intimacy, even if they do not exactly reproduce the experiences you had prior to prostate cancer treatments.

Whether or not you are planning to have sexual intercourse, some of the following treatments may prove helpful in restoring or improving erections.

## Oral Medications

Erection-enhancing drugs (PDE5i), such as tadalafil (Cialis), vardenafil (Levitra and Staxyn), and sildenafil (Viagra), are the most often tried medical treatment for erection problems following prostate cancer treatment. They need to be taken no less than one to two hours ahead of sexual activity. Sildenafil and vardenafil work over a four to six hour period. Tadalafil lasts in your system for up to 36 hours or more. While all of these PDE5i drugs can be taken daily, Cialis for daily use is formulated to maintain a steady level in your system so that you don't need to take a pill within an hour or two of engaging in sexual activity.

> High fat meals affect your body's absorption of Viagra, Staxyn, and Levitra. Don't eat a greasy, heavy meal, or you may find these pills do not work as well.

PDE5i drugs can help maintain good blood circulation in the penis independent of their specific use in aiding sexual activity, but they are more effective when coupled with physical and mental sexual stimulation. These drugs do not increase libido or change ejaculation or orgasm. They also may not be effective in men who have severe ED from either primary prostate cancer treatments or other diseases, such as diabetes.

PDE5i drugs should not be taken along with nitroglycerin (a medication for angina). They also are not recommended if you have:

- Decreased liver or kidney function.
- Very low or high blood pressure.
- Recently had a heart attack or stroke.
- Certain eye disorders such as glaucoma.

It is important to discuss with your doctor whether a PDE5i drug, or any drug, is right for you.

You can consume alcohol with these medications; however, you should be aware that alcohol itself often interferes with sexual ability.

## Injections

Several medications can produce an erection when injected by a fine needle into one side of the shaft of the penis. These often work better for men on ADT than oral medications because they are not as influenced by testosterone levels and sexual arousal. Although initially hesitant to use this form of treatment, many men find that they are able to administer the injections successfully with high satisfaction and little discomfort.

The most commonly used injectable medication is prostaglandin E1 (also known as alprostadil, and available as Caverject®, Edex®, and Prostin VR®). Other drugs are also used; phentolamine and papaverine can be blended by a pharmacist to form a combination commonly called "bimix," which may also be effective. Utilizing all three drugs (prostaglandin E1, papaverine, and phentolamine) is sometimes called "Triple P" or "trimix."

In order to inject these medications you need to have good visualization of the penis, so you may need a mirror or your partner to help.

If you use injections for erections and have an erection that lasts for more than three hours, go to the emergency room (ER) right away. Although an ER visit under these circumstances may be embarrassing, erections that last more than a few hours can lead to permanent injury to tissue in the penis from lack of oxygen. Most physicians suggest that injections should not be used more than three times a week.

### Intraurethral Suppositories

These small suppositories contain the medication prostaglandin E1 (sold as MUSE: Medicated Urethral System for Erection®). Instead of injecting the drug into the shaft of the penis, the MUSE system comes with a plastic applicator that places a small pellet of medication directly inside of the urethra. These suppositories are typically more effective when used with a constriction ring that is placed at the base of the shaft of the penis in order to keep the blood contained in the penis. For anatomical reasons, intraurethral suppositories are typically not as effective as penile injections.

> "I went into the exam room with a pretty high degree of apprehension, I mean, who really WANTS to stick a needle in the side of their penis?
>
> … Looking down, I was in complete disbelief about what I was about to do. I was shaking a little, but I just did it. After a small bit of resistance it went right in! I was shocked that I felt almost nothing, it honestly felt like a mosquito bite."–JD1969, cancerforums.net

> If you have a bleeding condition or are on blood thinners, such as Warfarin, penis rings and pumps are not recommended. They may increase your risk of bruising.

### Vacuum Pump

A vacuum erection device (VED) is a cylinder-shaped external pump that can be placed over the flaccid penis, using a lubricant to create a seal between the cylinder and the skin. These come with either a hand- or battery-powered pump that removes the air from the cylinder. This creates a vacuum around the penis. The lowered pressure draws blood into the shaft of the penis, making it swell and become firm. Once the penis is enlarged and firm, a rubber retaining ring is slipped onto the base of the penis to retain the blood in the shaft of the penis. The pump can then be removed. Battery-operated pumps may work better if your hand dexterity is poor, but in general, the hand-operated pumps create a stronger vacuum. After the constriction ring is in place, it should only remain on for about 30 minutes. Rings left on for hours can damage the tissue of the penis. The VED can be used safely on a daily basis.

A problem with erections produced by the VED is that only the shaft, and not the root of the penis, which lies inside the body, is engorged with blood. In natural unassisted erections, it is the engorged root of the penis that anchors the shaft and keeps the erection at the right angle for penile–vaginal sex. Erections obtained with the VED, though firm, tend to "swivel" at the base. This is known as the "hinge effect." Patients and their partners should be aware of this hinge effect since penetrative sex with erections from the VED may require manual assistance for insertion and some adjustment of posture to prevent separation during intercourse.

### Inflatable Penile Prosthesis (IPP)

The IPP is a bionic system, with inflatable cylinders surgically implanted into the shaft of the penis. The reservoir for fluid to fill the cylinders lies in the body cavity, and a small mechanical pump and valve lie in the scrotum. This hardware gives the man the option of having an erect penis for sexual activity and then a flaccid penis the rest of the time. The penis does not deflate after sexual activity until the man himself activates a release valve that lies in the scrotum and squeezes the fluid out of the cylinders. IPP devices are not visually detectable by others except for the small surgical scars where the hardware has been inserted. Once this procedure is done, it cannot be reversed. The IPP is an expensive option and is not always covered by insurance.

### Videos about Erectile Assistive Aids

If you have access to the Internet, the website Phoenix 5 for prostate cancer survivors has several videos showing how various medical treatments for erection problems work: phoenix5.org/menuvideos.html. Another option is www.aboutmen.ca/mens-health where you will find videos and explanations on how to give penile injections and use the VED, as well as discussions about penile prostheses. There are many other online resources about these ED treatments accessible through YouTube that you may find useful. Use the search terms "prostate cancer and sex" or "erectile dysfunction."

One couple, with great hesitancy, decided to try an ED treatment we recommended—something they had never done before. The wife reported back to us that while the treatment itself did not work, the process of experimenting with the treatment led them both to giggle and laugh a lot together— and in the process they shared a new and intimate experience that made them feel closer to each other than before they had tried it.

## Sex: Beyond Intercourse

Many men with a reduced ability to have erections and intercourse are worried that they won't be able to sexually satisfy their partner without penetration. Penetration and/or sexual intercourse are often seen as the essential part of sexuality for couples. Yet sexual activity can be understood as the expression of erotic love and physical affection between two individuals for the purposes of sexual arousal, pleasure, or connection. It may involve a variety of acts, not just penile–vaginal intercourse or anal sex, and most couples include a variety of types of touching and caressing as part of their lovemaking.

Activities that we typically think of as foreplay—for example, sexual talk, kissing, hugging, cuddling, sensual touching, genital touching, and oral sex—can be pleasurable in and of themselves, and can also lead to orgasm. It is okay not to orgasm every time, or even at all, with sexual activity. (Women seem to agree with this more easily than men.) That doesn't mean lovemaking has to be any less intimate or that it cannot be pleasurable. Sometimes, it is the pressure to reach orgasm that takes the pleasure out of sex.

When an erection problem makes penetration impossible, many couples give up on all sexual activity. Others continue to make love in other ways. Couples who have good communication skills and have used a variety of types of touch in their lovemaking prior to ADT are more likely to have a rewarding sexual life without intercourse.

Consider more foreplay, including using hand or oral methods of pleasuring one another. If you wish to try using fingers for vaginal penetration, make sure your nails are short, clean, and smooth. You may both find this to be a rewarding alternative to penile-vaginal intercourse. Women and men can experience orgasm without any penetration, and even if neither of you experience orgasm, foreplay can be pleasurable in and of itself.

If you have never tried giving oral sex before, now may be a good time to consider it. Oral sex can be great for both foreplay and climaxing. You may want to vary the ways in which you stimulate your partner (orally or manually) if you want to bring your partner to orgasm. In particular, women need several minutes before reaching orgasm and you may become fatigued. Provide reassuring messages to your partner about how you enjoy giving pleasure,—being in the right mindset will put your partner at ease and improve the experience. If your partner feels uncomfortable, or senses that you are uncomfortable, the experience may be less enjoyable. If this is the case, it may be best to try this lovemaking in small doses (a minute or two at a time) until it becomes more familiar to both of you.

### Suggestions for Pleasing Your Male Partner

Many men can reach orgasm with oral sex without having an erection.

One evening while you and your partner are on the couch or in bed, you may want to try this. First, take his hand and kiss his fingers. If he feels comfortable with that, take one of his fingers in your mouth and suck on it like a lollipop. You may see him getting aroused, or at least curious. If he seems to be enjoying this, consider going further. Unzip his pants and begin with kissing or licking the penis. When you feel ready, take the tip of his penis into your mouth. You may wish to try sucking on it, much like a vacuum. Communicate with your partner to find out what his preferences might be and where his hot spots are. If you are worried about ejaculate at orgasm, you need not; men who have had their prostates removed will not have any ejaculate at orgasm. Men on ADT, even if they still have their prostate, will also have no or very little ejaculate.

## Suggestions for Pleasing Your Female Partner

The majority of women say it is easier to reach orgasm when orally or manually stimulated than through intercourse.

Consider trying this. Kiss your partner's thighs and tummy, slowly working your way toward her genitals. The clitoris is located toward the top of the vulva, between the labial folds of skin and above the vaginal opening and urethra. It becomes engorged as a woman becomes aroused and is highly sensitive to stimulation; therefore, gently touching here can provide great pleasure. Try kissing the clitoris, and using your fingers to provide gentle stimulation in a circular motion. Try using your tongue in an up-and-down motion on the clitoris. Pay attention to your partner's response (e.g., changes in breathing, movement toward or away from you). Try asking your partner if what you are doing feels good, or if she might like softer or firmer pressure. You may want to try inserting a finger into the vagina while providing oral stimulation. Touching your partner's hips, waist, or breasts while providing oral stimulation is another option.

## The Use of Lubricants for Men and Women

With a full erection, stimulation of the sensory nerves in the penis is relatively easy (i.e., the nerves in the skin can be compressed against the firmer tissue below). However, without an erection it is more difficult to stimulate those nerves. Consequently, to produce pleasurable feeling and arousal, more pressure and stimulation must be applied to the penis, and for a longer period of time. As a result, there can be irritation of the skin. This can be painful and distracting, so lubrication is essential to avoid discomfort during extended penile stimulation.

In most drugstores and supermarkets, you can purchase lubricants that can be used for sexual activity. Some are warming, others are flavored, and others double as massage lotions.

- Water-based lubricants make for easier cleanup and may contain glycerine. *Examples:* K-Y® Liquid, Slippery Stuff®, Liquid Silk™, Astroglide®, or Dream Brands® The Natural. If using sex toys, a water-based lubricant is best for preserving the life of such products.

- Silicone- and oil-based lubricants are also available, last longer, and don't contain glycerine. Some couples prefer to use natural products as lubricants, such as coconut oil or olive oil.
- Petroleum-based lubricants such as Vaseline® are not recommended because they can promote bladder and vaginal infection.
- If your partner is a woman who has undergone menopause and you are engaging in penetrative activities, pick a lubricant that will not irritate her vaginal tissues. Clear, water-soluble, nonflavored lubricants are a good way to start.

**What activities involve pleasure and sensuality without penetrative intercourse?**

Hugging, cuddling, sharing passionate kisses, caressing, touching each other's erogenous zones, showing your partner where you want to be touched, kissing your partner's body, stimulating your partner with your fingers or tongue.

If you have never talked with your partner about some of these activities, now is a good time to ask what he or she might enjoy or be willing to try.

### Developing New Sexual Practices

One woman assumed that her partner no longer desired her and that engaging in any type of sexual activity was a burden and a chore for him. However, when she expressed this feeling to her partner, he assured her that while it might take more effort for him to want to engage in anything sexual, he still loved and desired her and took pleasure in being physically close to her. Through their discussion she learned that he was willing to try to please her, including doing what was necessary to sexually satisfy her even if he was not as sexually aroused as he used to be. Satisfying her was important for his need for intimacy too, and made him feel close to her.

It is common to believe that we know what our partner wants, particularly if we have been together for many years. However, often what our partner wants and what we want changes over the years, and can even change from day to day. Some sexual activities, which may have once been very important to you, may not be as important now...regardless of the influence of ADT. Similarly, you may think your partner is no longer interested in sexual activity when in fact he or she may still be in some ways. You may even surprise yourself; activities you never predicted you would like, you may now enjoy. Communicating about how important specific sexual activities are to each of you, and what you each find sensual and pleasuring, can help you recognize inaccurate assumptions or beliefs you may hold. This is an important step toward correcting those assumptions and achieving fulfilling intimate experiences.

### Activity: Mindfulness Exercise

One way to cultivate sexual experiences that focus on sensual touch is to practice mindful awareness. All too often we live our lives without being truly aware of our environment or what is going on in our bodies. Mindful awareness exercises help to develop skills focusing on physical sensations. Increasing your awareness of sensations and your ability to focus on sensation can help in your enjoyment of sensual or sexual pleasure. While initially you may practice this exercise on an individual basis, you can use this same exercise to tune into physical sensations while you are engaging sexually with your partner (as mentioned above). For more on the practice of mindfulness, see the Resources section (p. 135).

This exercise is designed to heighten awareness of your moment-by-moment experience and to become more in touch with the present. Consider practicing this technique when engaging in sensual touching with your partner. You can practice the exercise at the same time lying next to each other or have one partner focus on the exercise while the other gently touches. If your mind wanders during this exercise, this is fine; just bring your attention back to the activity at hand. Make sure you are seated comfortably, with your back against your chair and your feet placed on the ground. Or you can try this exercise lying down. Close your eyes if that is comfortable.

1. Begin by paying attention to your breath. Don't try to change it in any way; just start to bring awareness to your breathing. Pay attention to how your chest expands when you breathe in and how it falls as you breathe out. Notice the sensation of the air as it passes into and out of your nostrils each time you inhale and exhale. If that is uncomfortable for you, try breathing in through your nose and out through your mouth.
2. Begin to check in with your five senses. What do you hear? Can you label what those noises or distractions are? Can you taste or smell anything? If you do smell something, have you judged it to be positive or negative?
3. Begin to tune into your bodily sensations. Can you feel anything going on in your body? Can you feel your pulse? Is your stomach grumbling? Do you have an itch? Acknowledge these sensations.
4. Begin to become aware of your body's position in the chair or on the bed. Notice your legs and feet. Notice where your feet/legs contact the ground or bed. Take note of your thighs and buttocks and where they contact the surface beneath you. Notice how the surfaces hold the weight of your body. If you are sitting, check your posture to make sure that your head is well

supported either by the back of the chair or your neck. Find a comfortable position that allows the muscles in the back of your neck to relax.

5. Shift your attention to your hands. Are your hands resting on an armrest? Are they on your lap? Are they resting beside your body? Take note of where your hands are resting. What do they feel? Can your hands feel a certain texture? Is it rough or smooth? Soft or firm? Are they a certain temperature? Warm or cold?

6. Do you have any urges to move, change position, to become more comfortable? If so, scratch an itch, or adjust your posture accordingly; however, be conscious of your choice to do this, rather than just responding to the body in an automatic fashion. Be intentional in your motions, as you move your body.

7. When you feel ready, bring your attention back to the room and to your environment. Notice how refreshed and peaceful you feel, ready to carry on with the day.

We recommend that patients and family distressed about cancer look into a short course on mindful meditation. Increasingly, hospitals that treat cancer patients and other health care centers are offering such courses.

> Exercise and eating well help to maintain/improve sexual function by improving blood flow and nerve stimulation. When you feel healthy, your sexual self-esteem and energy improve from the mental boost and improved physical feeling. Furthermore just prior to sexual activity, you may want to take these tips into consideration before you decide to pursue sex:
> * Limit alcohol intake before making love.
> * Be well-rested.
> * Don't eat a huge meal directly beforehand.
> * Try to be present in the moment and enjoy the sensations you are experiencing.

## Activity: Beliefs Awareness

People often have unfounded beliefs about themselves and their sexual relationships with others. For example, a man may assume that a woman will leave him if he cannot sexually satisfy her through penile–vaginal intercourse. This can be a devastating assumption for a man who is experiencing reduced libido and ED due to ADT. Similarly, if patients lose interest in sex, partners may assume that they are no longer loved or desired. Beliefs or assumptions such as these can leave men on ADT and their intimate partners feeling isolated and depressed.

As a first key step toward maintaining intimacy in the face of ADT, it helps to be aware of your assumptions and discuss them with your partner. Often confronting an assumption and then challenging it, or having your partner challenge it, can clarify what is truly going on.

Here are two examples:

**Belief:**
*My partner has no libido when around me because he no longer loves and desires me.*

**Challenging that Belief:**
*My partner may no longer become sexually aroused, but he still loves spending time with me. He likes being physically intimate with me, even if that intimacy is not sexual.*

**Belief:**
*As a man, if I can't have erections, I can't please my partner.*

**Challenging that Belief:**
*I can ask my partner what his/her needs are and how to please him/her in other ways, either physically or sexually, for example, through sensual touch, massage, or oral sex.*

Think of some beliefs that you may have about yourself, your relationship with your partner, or your relationship with others once the effects of ADT begin. Then challenge each belief in the spaces provided below. See the Appendix for an additional copy (p. 130).

**Belief:** _____

**Challenge:** _____

_____

_____

**Belief:** _____

**Challenge:** _____

_____

_____

## Using Sexual Aids and Sex Toys

It has become increasingly common for couples to include "sex toys" in their sexual activities, whether or not ED or changes in libido are affecting their relationship. Using sex toys may or may not be a new idea for you and your partner. The use of such toys may help lengthen your sexual interaction by saving your energy since you will not have to stimulate your partner manually for as long. There are a variety of such sex toys available, including *vibrators*, which come in many sizes and for many purposes, and *dildos*, which are used for penetration.

> Some men on ADT have told us that they discovered, to their surprise, that with stimulation to the penis through a vibrator, and with enough desire, they can reach orgasm, though they had previously thought it was impossible.

The main feature of a vibrator, as the name suggests, is that it provides stimulation through vibration. Small vibrators can be used to focus on clitoral stimulation, and other vibrators can be used to insert into the vagina to stimulate the "G-spot." There are vibrators designed specifically for men to place around the head of the penis where the nerve endings are most sensitive. Some products are relatively inexpensive, such as the Wahl® vibrator with the cup attachment. The Viberect®, which has double paddles, is specifically marketed for men with ED; however, it is very pricey, and there are no published data to show that it is superior to two simpler and cheaper vibrators used together. Vibrators can also be used anally for male or female stimulation, and some vibrators can be looped around the penis to stimulate both the clitoris and the testicles at the same time.

There are several types of dildos that can be used for vaginal or anal penetration. They come in a variety of materials including silicone, metal, and glass.

> An experienced sales person at a popular sex shop told us that what she likes most about her job is that couples who come into the store are invariably curious and upbeat, never unhappy.

Always buy high-quality sex toys that are visibly new. Be sure to clean sex toys before each use. There is some concern about the chemicals in soft toys, so if you purchase them, consider covering them with a condom. If you have any allergies, such as to latex, ensure that your toys are hypoallergenic and that you don't use oil-based lubricants with them. You should not use a silicone lubricant with a silicone sex toy, as it will erode the toy. Don't be too rough with toys; be careful not to insert too deeply or forcefully.

An alternative to ED treatments is for a male to use a strap-on dildo to penetrate his partner. A harness is worn on the man's hips, which holds a penis-like dildo in essentially the same position that an erect penis would be. When the partner reaches down and stimulates the patient's penis with a lubricated hand while the patient thrusts with the strap-on, many patients have reported that it feels exactly as if their penis is inside their partner and that it is easy to reach orgasm. Patients report relief knowing that they don't have to fear losing an erection during sexual activity or disappointing their partner. Consequently, both patients and partners have reported that they enjoy this sexual aid. One company, SpareParts®, makes a harness specifically for males, called the Deuce®, which can be purchased in several different sizes from many of the larger sex shops in North America.

If the idea of sex toys is awkward or intimidating to you, consider experimenting with simpler things. You can start out with massage oils, feathers, and other erotic touch products that you may not have used before, eventually experiment with a sexual aid such as a vibrator, and progress from there. The best way to approach the use of sex toys is to have an open mind and not be afraid to laugh if it doesn't go as well as you expected. Sometimes just experimenting with something new with your partner can bring you both closer together. Just talking about such options and shopping together (in stores or online) for sex aids can help a couple build intimacy.

> Some of the benefits of incorporating toys into your sex play may include experiencing excitement associated with trying something new and different, discovering the capacity for a new kind of penetrative intercourse (e.g., use of a hand-held or strap-on dildo), and avoiding fatigue during extended stimulation by using vibrators.

### Activity: Pros/Cons Table · · · · · · · · · · · · · · · · · ·

If you have been reading through this book chapter by chapter, you should be familiar with the value of the Pros/Cons exercise by now. This exercise can be applied to any decision you are thinking about making in your life. Here is an example as it may relate to addressing sexual intimacy.

|  | PROS | CONS |
| --- | --- | --- |
| **MAKING THE CHANGE:** <br> Try engaging in nonpenetrative sexual activity | • Remain sexually connected with my partner <br><br> • Provide pleasure to my partner <br><br> • Enjoy receiving pleasure myself | • It might make me sad to compare what we used to have with what we can do now |
| **STAYING THE SAME:** <br> Don't have sex until my erections come back | • Don't have to focus on what I have lost <br><br> • Avoid feeling like a failure when I can't get an erection | • My partner and I may feel disconnected |

Now, try it out for yourself.

|  | PROS | CONS |
|---|---|---|
| **MAKING THE CHANGE:** | | |
| | | |
| | | |
| **STAYING THE SAME:** | | |
| | | |
| | | |

## Activity: Action Plan

In the previous chapter you were introduced to an Action Plan on page 78. Again you are reminded that it is best to start small with something very manageable (e.g., arranging a date night) before you take on larger-scale goals (e.g., using an erectile aid for sexual intercourse). You may wish to place your action plan in a location where you will see it regularly throughout your day.

### Action Plan Example: Increasing Physical Affection

**What I plan to do:** show my partner more physical affection

**When I plan to do it:** give her a kiss and hug in the morning when I leave for work and when I get home; go to bed 15 minutes earlier than usual so we can cuddle in bed before we go to sleep

**Who I might do it with:** my partner

**Why my plan is important:** to help her feel appreciated, loved, and prioritized

**Where I plan to do it:** in my home

**What might get in the way?** forgetting

**How I will address what might get in the way:** I will tell my partner my plan so she can be more affectionate with me too, which will remind me.

On the facing page is a blank copy that you can fill out. An additional copy is located in the Appendix (p. 124). It helps to be as specific as possible.

**Action Plan:** _____

What I plan to do: _____

_____

When I plan to do it: _____

_____

Who I might do it with: _____

_____

Why my plan is important: _____

_____

Where I plan to do it: _____

_____

What might get in the way? _____

_____

How I will address what might get in the way: _____

_____

## Activity: Goal Setting and Confidence

In order to support your goal, take a moment to rate the following factors associated with your goal. First, write down your goal (this might be what you have written in your Action Plan):

**Goal** _____

i) Rate how confident you feel that you'll achieve your goal:

| 1 | 2 | 3 | 4 | 5 | 6 | 7 | 8 | 9 | 10 |
|---|---|---|---|---|---|---|---|---|---|

Not confident                                                    Very confident

ii) Rate how motivated you are to accomplish your goal:

| 1 | 2 | 3 | 4 | 5 | 6 | 7 | 8 | 9 | 10 |
|---|---|---|---|---|---|---|---|---|---|

Not motivated                                                    Very motivated

iii) Rate how likely you are to actually carry out your goal:

| 1 | 2 | 3 | 4 | 5 | 6 | 7 | 8 | 9 | 10 |
|---|---|---|---|---|---|---|---|---|---|

Not likely                                                          Very likely

If any of your answers *are less than 5*:

• Some ways to enhance motivation: (a) Enlist the help of your partner to hold you accountable, (b) Set up a reward system so that when you have achieved the goal, you can reward yourself, (c) Review a list of the possible benefits that may come from this change in behavior.

• If your confidence rating is really low, consider revising your goal—is it too ambitious? Can you start with a more modest goal and work your way up to a more significant lifestyle change?

• If you're at a 2, 3, or 4, for any of the questions, remind yourself of the reason you chose that number and not a zero—what are the reasons why you are motivated to make this change?

• Another strategy is to consider completing the previous Pros/Cons table to help you identify your motivations (pros) for making this change, but also some of the barriers (cons) that might be getting in the way of making the change.

### Effects on Intimate Relationships and Sexuality: Essentials

ADT will probably influence the sexual and intimate aspects of your relationship as a couple. Most men (approximately 90%) on ADT experience a reduced libido, leading to less frequent desire, or no desire, for sexual activities. This can be a source of relief for some couples and can cause significant distress for others. You may need to discuss what sex means to you and to your partner, and how the two of you will adjust to this change. Specifically, how might you maintain physical closeness if sexual activity is no longer the prominent physical interaction between you? The exercises in this chapter may help you plan ahead and decide what is important to you.

Even with a reduced libido, it is possible to find sexual pleasure and sensuality. As a couple, you can redefine your sexual activities to include activities other than penetrative (i.e., penile–vaginal or anal) sex. You can explore new or forgotten sexual activities. The partner who, previous to ADT, may have been less responsible for initiation can become more expressive and be the one to initiate sensual activities. You can make the commitment to sample sensual and pleasurable activities without pressure to achieve erection, intercourse, or orgasm. The mere act of jointly planning the time and location for these intimate and enjoyable activities can help maintain an intimate bond. Together, you can practice sensual touch or try activities to stimulate your appetite for physical intimacy and sensuality.

We encourage you to explore physical closeness beyond erection-dependent sexual activities. With an open mind, a commitment to each other, and a willingness to co-explore, physical intimacy can be rewarding even without it leading to penetrative intercourse. Sexual activity need not require an erection or lead to orgasm for it to be a pleasing and bonding experience for both partners. The key to all of this is communication with each other about your expectations and willingness to explore.

### Moving Forward: Questions for Discussion

Starting conversations about sexuality is often very difficult. The following questions for couples to ask each other may help to initiate communication and clarify expectations about sexual activities:

- Are you comfortable with one of us reaching orgasm even if the other does not?
- How do you feel about us touching, caressing, and cuddling without either of us reaching or attempting to reach orgasm?
- What do you think about us acquiring a sex toy to use in our sex play?

The patient may want to ask his partner:

- What should we do when you get aroused and I don't?
- Is it okay if I bring you to orgasm through touching or oral caressing even though I no longer have full erections?
- How do you feel about me using or exploring erectile aids and/or sex toys?

The partner may want to ask the patient:

- Do you still enjoy me touching you even though you don't get fully sexually aroused?
- What kinds of touching do you most enjoy now?

## NOTES:

_____

_____

_____

_____

_____

_____

# 7

# Impact on Committed Relationships

Partners of men on ADT sometimes report that they do not know how to communicate about the changes that are occurring within their relationship. Those who neglect to communicate with each other can become isolated. Those who feel they must hide their feelings and emotional changes, not only from each other but also from others, may withdraw from friends and social networks.

Men who feel closest to their partners during sexual activity may nevertheless withdraw from them when their sex drive is diminished by ADT. The couple may talk less because the patient no longer feels close to his partner. This can leave the partner feeling less wanted, less desired, or less attractive. These losses can be traumatic to each individual, and to the couple as a whole. For example, one patient told us: "Not having a good sex life really made me withdraw. I wasn't even going to touch her because she would think I would be interested when I'm really not, and then she might get all hot and bothered and I'm not ..."

In sharp contrast, there are other couples who find that they actually connect more with each other because the experience of having cancer has brought them closer together. Some report that after many years together, they were perfectly fine with no longer having penetrative sex and yet were still able to maintain true intimacy in their relationship.

Most people find it important to feel genuinely understood by their partner and to know they can talk about things, even things that stir up strong emotions. Initiating a discussion on emotionally sensitive topics can be a challenge at first, but can help increase a couple's confidence that they can face whatever new challenges lay ahead. Yet, as the partner of an ADT patient describes below, verbal communication is not the only way to share your feelings.

> "We take such comfort in [talking], yet we can undo everything we've said in one gesture or in one look, or even in one misinterpretation. Show me. Take me outside and let's watch the sunset together. Put your arm around me and pull me to your side for a long hug that tells me I'm treasured. ... Touch me, even if it's just a gentle hand on my shoulder, or on my leg beneath the table. ... ease off at the first sign of resistance. I will do the same, always respecting the signals you give, whether you utter them or not. Show me. Discover me. Rediscover us. Show me what you are saying is true. Then I'll listen to what you need to say."
>
> —Partner/caregiver as quoted in "Intimacy Challenged by Surgery, Radiation, or ADT" by Charles (Chuck) Maack (www.theprostateadvocate.com)

## Potential Changes in the Relationship

### Changes in the Way You Interact With Each Other

It is possible that during or after ADT, partners may change the ways in which they relate to each other, and even change the activities that they engage in together at home. Some couples dealing with cancer report being able to draw closer to each other, finding new appreciation for their relationship. Other couples dealing with ADT say that because they are unable to maintain a high level of sexual intimacy they have started to drift apart; they live in the same house, but put on an act of being married. One or both partners may come to resent the other for the changes that are occurring in themselves and in their relationship. To better understand the impact of ADT in your own relationship, consider reflecting with your partner on the ways you relate to each other, and how your relationship may or may not change if you as a couple become less sexually active after beginning ADT.

Different couples respond to the changes brought on by ADT in various ways, and some couples find adapting to change easier than other couples. The box at left presents one couple's story of drifting apart.

We hope that you can avoid ending up like this couple. The goal in bringing this story to your attention is to encourage you as a couple to think about and discuss ways to reduce the stress from ADT so you can remain close to each other and avoid drifting apart.

### Increased Self-Doubt

Both the patient and his partner may experience increased self-doubt or decreased confidence when faced with the changes that ADT introduces to their lives. Either person may begin to question if the partner still sees him or

> "The problems were solved when one day I moved into another room. I have my own bathroom, and I take care of my own affairs without involving my wife. It isn't the way I thought things would turn out, but it's preferable to endless quarrels and divorce, and my wife seems to be content. ... We discuss practical matters without drifting into feelings, and when friends and family visit we put on a performance of intimacy and unity."
>
> —Prostate cancer patient, as quoted in Navon and Morag, 2003

It is important to recognize that a man on ADT is less likely to spontaneously touch his partner, and that this can be devastating to the partner.

You can do simple things to let your partner know that you still care and find him or her desirable. Make a point of telling your partner directly that you find him or her attractive and desirable. Do special things for each other (e.g., make a meal, write a love letter) that express how you feel. Spending quality time together and making a conscious effort to maintain physical contact and sensuality can help both of you overcome self-doubt and avoid drifting apart.

Increased effort to display physical but nonsexual affection, and increased effort in letting your partner know in visible ways that you care for him or her, can help to make up for and even overcome reduced sexual activity.

herself as attractive and desirable. Most people feel confident and attractive, when they are able to sexually arouse their partner—and this could become an issue when ADT leads to reduced libido.

Bear in mind that attraction and desire are not limited to sexual activities. We encourage you to openly reaffirm to each other that you appreciate each other's company, closeness, and intimacy, both of a sexual and a nonsexual nature.

If you neglect to do this, you or your partner may withdraw from the relationship and your communication and intimate bond might be damaged. If you doubt yourself and your relationship, it may make the transition to living with ADT, and managing ADT side effects in particular, even more challenging.

> "We show each other affection; we're cuddling and having our kisses. We're just there for each other ... we do love each other. We have our hugs. We have our laughs."—Adam, patient

Therefore, after the patient is on ADT, it is important that each of you make a concerted effort to let your partner know that you still care about him or her and desire closeness, even if spontaneous and unassisted penetrative sex is no longer possible.

One patient told us that he made his partner feel special by doing things for her that she knows require some sacrifice on his part. He shared, "I love to make cabbage rolls for my partner even though I don't like to eat them myself."

Below are some of the things we hear from couples about why physical affection in general, and not just penetrative sex, is important to them. You may find some comments here that apply to you. Feel free to add your own thoughts to the list.

Physical affection with my partner:

- Calms me down.
- Helps me feel special.

* Makes me feel desired.
* Helps me feel close to my partner.
* Reminds me that my partner is here for me.

_____

_____

_____

## Activity: Pros/Cons Table

If you have been reading previous chapters of this book, you should be familiar with the value of the Pros/Cons table by now. This exercise can be applied to any decision you are thinking about making in your life. Here is an example as it may relate to addressing sexual intimacy.

|  | PROS | CONS |
|---|---|---|
| **MAKING THE CHANGE:** Show more physical affection to my partner | • Physical affection helps my partner to feel appreciated <br><br> • Hugs and kisses keep us physically and emotionally connected | • Requires effort to remind myself to show her more affection <br><br> • Might feel artificial |
| **STAYING THE SAME:** Stop being physically affectionate | • Prevents a misunderstanding that my partner might think I am interested in sex when I'm not | • We may become more disconnected <br><br> • She might interpret my lack of physical affection as not being interested in her |

Now, try it out for yourself.

|  | PROS | CONS |
|---|---|---|
| **MAKING THE CHANGE:** |  |  |
| **STAYING THE SAME:** |  |  |

## Activity: Action Plan

In the previous chapters you were introduced to the value of an Action Plan. Again you are reminded that it is best to start small with something very manageable (e.g., walking regularly) before you take on larger scale goals (e.g., running a 10-km race). Hang your completed form somewhere where you will see it every day, like next to your bathroom mirror or on your fridge, to remind yourself of your commitment to this goal.

### Action Plan Example: Communicate More Effectively With My Partner

**What I plan to do:** have a conversation once about ADT-related changes

**When I plan to do it:** Sunday mornings when we go for breakfast

**Who I might do it with:** my partner

**Why my plan is important:** to make sure that we talk about things explicitly to prevent misunderstandings and prevent avoidance of discussing important topics due to discomfort

**Where I plan to do it:** at the local café and deli

**What might get in the way?** anxiety about the conversation

**How I will address what might get in the way:** I will tell my partner, so they can appropriately support me.

Here is a blank copy that you can fill out. An additional copy is located in the Appendix on page 124. It helps to be as specific as possible when you are making your Action Plan.

**Action Plan:** _____

What I plan to do: _____

_____

When I plan to do it: _____

_____

Who I might do it with: _____

_____

Why my plan is important: _____

_____

Where I plan to do it: _____

_____

What might get in the way? _____

_____

How I will address what might get in the way: _____

_____

### Activity: Goal Setting and Confidence

A strategy that can help you in accomplishing your goal is to take a moment to rate the following factors: confidence, motivation, and predicted likelihood of completion. First, write down your goal (this may be what you wrote in your Action Plan):

**Goal:** _____

i) Rate how confident you feel that you'll achieve your goal:

| 1 | 2 | 3 | 4 | 5 | 6 | 7 | 8 | 9 | 10 |

Not confident                                                Very confident

ii) Rate how motivated you are to accomplish your goal:

| 1 | 2 | 3 | 4 | 5 | 6 | 7 | 8 | 9 | 10 |

Not motivated                                          Very motivated

iii) Rate how likely you are to actually carry out your goal:

| 1 | 2 | 3 | 4 | 5 | 6 | 7 | 8 | 9 | 10 |

Not likely                                              Very likely

If any of your answers *are less than 5*:

- Consider ways to enhance motivation, such as enlisting the help of your partner or a friend to hold you accountable or rewarding yourself with something you are looking forward to. For additional details regarding enhancing motivation and rewards see pages 42 to 43 in Chapter 3.
- Consider revising your goal—is it too ambitious? Can you start with a more modest goal and work your way up to a more significant lifestyle change?
- Remind yourself of the reasons why you're at a 2, 3, or 4, and not a zero—what are the reasons why you indicated that you were not at a zero?
- Consider completing the previous Pros/Cons table. This will help you identify your motivations (pros) for making this change, but also some of the barriers (cons) that might be getting in the way of making the change.

### Impact on Committed Relationships: Essentials

Individuals and couples react differently to the effects of ADT. Some couples will grow closer, and some couples will grow apart. Some couples may take on a role more like roommates rather than lovers. If it is of value for you as a couple to maintain the quality of the relationship you currently have, then you will have to plan ahead, preparing to adapt to change. However, each of you will react in your own way, so it is important to communicate openly about how you are feeling.

As the man's libido decreases with ADT and the nature of sexual contact is altered, self-doubt may occur. For example, you may wonder if your partner still finds you desirable or attractive, either in sexual or nonsexual ways. The danger of this is that you as a couple can fall into a trap of self-doubt, where one or both of you isolate yourselves, and you fail to communicate with each other. This further fuels self-doubt and compromises your relationship. It is important that you frequently let each other know, even in little and nonsexual ways, that you still care for and desire each other.

## Moving Forward: Questions for Discussion

The following are questions that can be helpful for partners to answer together:

- How do cancer and its treatment change the plans we had for our lives?
- How do we deal with the uncertainty of our future?
- In what ways do you feel different about me or yourself as a man/woman (e.g., abilities, roles, or dreams) now that we are facing a new cancer treatment?
- What have we lost—and what have we gained—through this experience so far?

Add your own questions here:

_____

_____

_____

_____

Then consider the following:

- How can I make sure that I let my partner know that I still love, desire, and cherish him/her even if ADT challenges our relationship?
- What are the things that make my partner feel most loved?
- What are the things that make me feel most loved?

**NOTES:**

# 8

# Conclusion: Staying Healthy

As you come to the end of this book, we want to emphasize and reiterate some of its major themes. ADT has substantial side effects that can negatively impact a person's quality of life. As you have read, there are both physical and psychological side effects of this treatment. Some of the side effects, such as reduced libido, impact not just the patient but also the dynamic of a couple's relationship. Managing ADT side effects can be a challenge for both the patient and those close to him.

Adapting to ADT and staying healthy while androgen-deprived can be best handled by both the patient and his partner being aware of the side effects and preemptively taking actions to deal with them. Managing the physical side effects may require a substantial commitment to changes in one's lifestyle (e.g., diet and exercise). Maintaining a healthy BMI (body mass index) and an active lifestyle may not be easy, but the benefits are well established and they are the most effective way to stay healthy while on ADT.

To deal with the psychological affects of ADT, particularly those that may be noticed by those closest to the patient, it helps to be aware of them and be willing to talk about them with others. To try to hide or deny them is neither helpful for the patient nor those he normally interacts with closely.

# Appendix

In this appendix you will find additional copies of these tools for change:

1. Drug Chart
2. PSA Chart
3. Hot Flash Diary
4. Pros/Cons Table
5. Action Plan
6. Goal Setting and Confidence
7. Side Effects Self-Assessment
8. Screening for Emotional Distress
9. Beliefs Awareness Exercise

## 1. Drug Chart

This chart can be used to document your specific medications for androgen deprivation therapy. For example, you might list the medication that you receive for your injections and how often you get your injection.

| Medication | Dose | How Often? |
|---|---|---|
| | | |
| | | |
| | | |
| | | |
| | | |
| | | |
| | | |
| | | |
| | | |

## 2. PSA Chart

This is a chart for you to use to track your PSA results.

| Date | PSA Level | Date | PSA Level | Date | PSA Level |
|------|-----------|------|-----------|------|-----------|
|      |           |      |           |      |           |
|      |           |      |           |      |           |
|      |           |      |           |      |           |
|      |           |      |           |      |           |
|      |           |      |           |      |           |
|      |           |      |           |      |           |
|      |           |      |           |      |           |
|      |           |      |           |      |           |
|      |           |      |           |      |           |
|      |           |      |           |      |           |

## 3. Hot Flash Diary

This exercise is an exercise to help you cope with bothersome hot flashes. The instructions for how to complete this exercise can be found on page 13.

| Day | Intensity (0–10) | Duration | Distressing Thought/ Appraisal | Coping Statement |
|---|---|---|---|---|
| Sunday | | | | |
| Monday | | | | |
| Tuesday | | | | |
| Wednesday | | | | |
| Thursday | | | | |
| Friday | | | | |
| Saturday | | | | |

## 4. Pros/Cons Table

Sometimes, even though you *want* to make a lifestyle change, you may need to persuade yourself that the change is in fact worthwhile. A Pros/Cons table is a great way to convince yourself, and you can redo it anytime you feel as if your life and priorities have shifted.

| | PROS | CONS |
|---|---|---|
| **MAKING THE CHANGE:** | | |
| **STAYING THE SAME:** | | |

## 5. Action Plan

Throughout the book there are suggestions for changes that will help you and your partner maintain a high quality of life while on ADT. An Action Plan is a structured way to help you be clear about your goals, and increase the likelihood that you will follow through on your plans.

Here are some blank copies that you can fill out. It helps to be as specific as possible when you are making your action plan. Specific examples are detailed in each chapter.

**ACTION PLAN:** _____

What I plan to do: _____

_____

When I plan to do it: _____

_____

Who I might do it with: _____

_____

Why my plan is important: _____

_____

Where I plan to do it: _____

_____

What might get in the way? _____

_____

How I will address what might get in the way: _____

_____

## 6. Goal Setting and Confidence

In order to support your goal, it can be helpful to ask yourself how confident you are that you can be successful in making this change.

First, write down your goal:

**Goal:** _____

(e.g., To start walking every day)

i) Rate how confident you feel that you'll achieve your goal:

1    2    3    4    5    6    7    8    9    10
Not confident                                    Very confident

ii) Rate how motivated you are to accomplish your goal:

1    2    3    4    5    6    7    8    9    10
Not motivated                                    Very motivated

iii) Rate how likely you are to actually carry out your goal:

1    2    3    4    5    6    7    8    9    10
Not likely                                       Very likely

If any of your answers *are less than 5*:

- Consider enlisting the help of your partner or a friend to hold you accountable.
- Consider revising your goal—is it too ambitious? Can you start with a more modest goal and work your way up to a more significant lifestyle change?
- Remind yourself of the reasons why you are motivated to make this change.

## 7. Side Effects Self-Assessment

For descriptions and management strategies of the side effects listed below, see the appropriate chapter.

1. *During the past month*, how often have you experienced hot flashes? (*Please circle one number*).
   (1) More than once a day
   (2) About once a day
   (3) More than once a week
   (4) About once a week
   (5) Rarely or never

2. *During the past month*, how often have you had breast tenderness/ sensitivity? (*Please circle one number*).
   (1) More than once a day
   (2) About once a day
   (3) More than once a week
   (4) About once a week
   (5) Rarely or never

3. *During the past month*, have you noticed any breast enlargement? (*Please circle one number*).
   (1) None
   (2) Minimal
   (3) Substantial
   (4) Moderate

4. *During the past month*, how much has your weight changed, if at all? (*Please circle one number*).
   (1) Gained 10 pounds/4.5 kilograms or more
   (2) Gained less than 10 pounds/4.5 kilograms
   (3) No change in weight
   (4) Lost less than 10 pounds/4.5 kilograms
   (5) Lost 10 pounds/4.5 or more kilograms or more

5. *During the past month*, have you experienced a change in the amount of hair on your arms, legs, and torso? (*Please circle one number*).
   (1) Loss of body hair on arms, legs, and/or torso
   (2) No loss of body hair

6. *During the past month*, how concerned have you been about changes in how your penis and scrotum look?
   (1) Not concerned
   (2) Moderately concerned
   (3) A little concerned
   (4) Highly concerned

7. *During the past month,* how has your level of sexual desire been? (*Please circle one number*).
   (1) Very low to none
   (2) Low
   (3) Moderate
   (4) High
   (5) Very high

8. *During the past month,* how has your ability to have an erection been? (*Please circle one number*).
   (1) Very poor to none
   (2) Poor
   (3) Fair
   (4) Good
   (5) Very good/Excellent

9. *During the past month,* how often have you experienced a problem remembering something that you thought you knew well? (*Please circle one number*).
   (1) More than once a day
   (2) About once a day
   (3) More than once a week
   (4) About once a week
   (5) Rarely or never

10. *During the past month,* how often have you felt depressed? (*Please circle one number*).
    (1) More than once a day
    (2) About once a day
    (3) More than once a week
    (4) About once a week
    (5) Rarely or never

11. *During the past month,* how often have you felt a lack of energy? (*Please circle one number*).
    (1) More than once a day
    (2) About once a day
    (3) More than once a week
    (4) About once a week
    (5) Rarely or never

## 8. Screening for Emotional Distress
## Mood Questionnaire

The following questionnaire (The Patient Health Questionnaire (PHQ-9)) is designed to assess different aspects of your mood. Indicate your response using the categories on the right.

**How often have you been experienced the following problems in the past two weeks?**

| | Not at All | Several Days | More Than Half the Days | Nearly Every Day |
|---|---|---|---|---|
| 1. Little interest or pleasure in doing things | 0 | 1 | 2 | 3 |
| 2. Feeling down, depressed, or hopeless | 0 | 1 | 2 | 3 |
| 3. Trouble falling asleep or staying asleep, or sleeping too much | 0 | 1 | 2 | 3 |
| 4. Feeling tired or having little energy | 0 | 1 | 2 | 3 |
| 5. Poor appetite or overeating | 0 | 1 | 2 | 3 |
| 6. Feeling bad about yourself, or that you are a failure, or that you have let yourself or your family down | 0 | 1 | 2 | 3 |
| 7. Trouble concentrating on things, such as reading the newspaper or watching television | 0 | 1 | 2 | 3 |
| 8. Moving or speaking so slowly that other people could have noticed. Or the opposite—being so fidgety or restless that you have been moving around a lot more than usual | 0 | 1 | 2 | 3 |
| 9. Thoughts that you would be better off dead or of hurting yourself in some way | 0 | 1 | 2 | 3 |
| **Column Totals:** | | ____ + | ____ + | ____ |
| **Add Column Totals Together:** | | _____ | | |

*Scoring Instructions:*
- Scores below 5 indicate no concern.
- Scores between 5 and 14 indicate some mild symptoms of difficulty with mood. You may be able to address these by seeking support from family and friends, beginning to work through a self-help book (see the Resources section on p. 135 for suggestions), or making efforts to engage in more rewarding and pleasurable activities in your life.
- Scores of 15 or higher indicate symptoms of depression and likely warrant seeking help from a professional counselor and/or family physician.

## Symptoms of Distress Questionnaire

The following questionnaire (Generalized Anxiety Disorder 7-Item (GAD-7) Scale) is designed to assess symptoms of distress. Using the categories on the right, indicate the most applicable answer for each item.

**How often have you been experienced the following problems in the past two weeks?**

| | Not at All | Several Days | More Than Half the Days | Nearly Every Day |
|---|---|---|---|---|
| 1. Feeling nervous, anxious, or on edge | 0 | 1 | 2 | 3 |
| 2. Not being able to stop or control worrying | 0 | 1 | 2 | 3 |
| 3. Worrying too much about different things | 0 | 1 | 2 | 3 |
| 4. Trouble relaxing | 0 | 1 | 2 | 3 |
| 5. Being so restless that it's hard to sit still | 0 | 1 | 2 | 3 |
| 6. Becoming easily annoyed or irritable | 0 | 1 | 2 | 3 |
| 7. Feeling afraid, as if something awful might happen | 0 | 1 | 2 | 3 |
| **Column Totals:** | | ___ + | ___ + | ___ |
| **Add Totals Together:** | | _____ | | |

*Scoring Instructions:*
- Scores below 5 indicate no concern.
- Scores between 5 and 10 indicate some mild symptoms of difficulty with stress. You may be able to address these by seeking support from family and friends, beginning to work through a self-help book (see the Resources section on p. 135 for suggestions), or practicing the relaxation exercises listed below
- Scores over 10 indicate symptoms of anxiety and warrant seeking help from a professional counselor and/or family physician.

## 9. Beliefs Awareness Exercise

The instructions for this exercise can be found on page 98–99.

**Belief:** _____

**Challenge:** _____

_____

_____

**Belief:** _____

**Challenge:** _____

_____

_____

**Belief:** _____

**Challenge:** _____

_____

_____

**Belief:** _____

**Challenge:** _____

_____

_____

# Glossary

**ADT**—Androgen deprivation therapy, also known as hormone therapy; a therapy designed to inhibit the body's production of androgens, testosterone in particular.

> **ADT2**—ADT where the patient takes both an LHRH drug and also an antiandrogen drug. *See also* ADT.

> **ADT3**—ADT where the patient takes concurrently an LHRH drug, an antiandrogen drug, and a 5-alpha-reductase inhibitor. *See also* ADT.

**Antiandrogen**—Drugs that prevent androgens from activating cells. Antiandrogens do this by competing with natural androgens for the appropriate receptors on the cells and blocking those receptors so that natural androgens can't activate them. *See also* Androgen.

**Androgen**—Any substance, such as testosterone or dihydrotestosterone, that promotes male characteristics (e.g., body hair).

**Brachytherapy**—Treatment with ionizing radiation where the radiation source is inserted directly into the target organ, usually in the form of small seeds or pellets.

**Castration**—Removal of the testicles by surgery or making them inactive by chemical means so they cannot produce sperm or testosterone. Chemical and surgical castrations are equally effective in lowering testosterone levels. *See also* ADT, Orchiectomy.

**Cognitive function**—An intellectual process by which one becomes aware of, perceives, or comprehends ideas. It involves all aspects of perception, thinking, reasoning, and remembering.

**CT**—A computed tomography (CT) scan creates images of the body by using x-rays.

**Dihydrotestosterone (DHT)**—A natural androgen that is more potent than testosterone. It is produced in the body from testosterone by the enzyme 5-alpha reductase. *See also* Testosterone.

**Erectile dysfunction (ED)**—Inability of a man to maintain an erection sufficient for satisfying sexual penetration.

**Estradiol**—The most potent naturally occurring estrogen found in both males and females. *See also* Estrogen.

**Estrogen**—Any of several steroid hormones that are secreted primarily by the ovaries and placenta in females and promote development of female secondary sex characteristics (e.g., breasts). In males the primary estrogen is estradiol and it is normally made from testosterone by the enzyme aromatase. *See also* Hormones.

**GnRH antagonists**—Also called LHRH antagonists. Synthetic (man-made) hormones that block a chemical signal from the brain to the **pituitary gland** at the base of the brain. That, in turn, stops the release from the pituitary gland the hormones that "tell" the testes to make **testosterone**. *See also* LHRH agonists, Hormones.

**Gynecomastia**—Enlargement of the breast tissue in males.

**Hormones**—Hormones are compounds in the body that are produced by endocrine glands and have specific target tissues in the body. They activate or suppress activity in their target tissue. Hormones can be internally secreted or pharmaceutically produced.

**IU**—International Units

**LHRH Agonists**—A synthetic (man-made) hormone that binds to receptors in the pituitary gland. This first causes a rise in normal signals from the pituitary gland to the testes to make testosterone. This leads to a feedback loop, which then shuts down the signal to the pituitary leading to a loss of the hormonal signal to the testes to produce testosterone. *See also* GnRH antagonists and hormones.

**Metabolic syndrome**—A condition associated with obesity, including elements such as glucose intolerance, insulin resistance, and raised blood pressure, which increases the risk of cardiovascular disease and diabetes.

**Orchiectomy**—Surgical removal of the testes. *See also* Castration.

**Osteoporosis**—A disorder in which the bones become increasingly porous, brittle, and subject to fracture, due to a loss of calcium and other mineral components. Osteoporotic fractures can lead to decreased height and skeletal deformities. Osteoporosis is common in older persons, primarily postmenopausal women, but also is associated with androgen deprivation from long-term LHRH agonist and GnRH antagonist use, or orchiectomy.

**Phosphodiesterase-5 inhibitors (PDE5i)**—Drugs used to treat erectile dysfunction. These include the oral drugs Viagra®, Cialis®, and Levitra®. *See also* Erectile dysfunction.

**Pituitary gland**—A structure attached by a stalk to the base of the brain, which controls many of the hormonal pathways in the body.

**Prostatectomy**—The surgical removal of part or all of the prostate gland.

**Prostate-specific antigen (PSA)**—A protein, produced by prostate cells, elevated levels of which may indicate the presence of prostate cancer or other prostatic disease. *See also* PSA test.

**PSA test**—A blood test that measures the amount of PSA in the serum. *See also* Prostate-specific antigen.

**Radiation therapy**—Use of high-energy, penetrating waves or particles such as x-rays, gamma rays, proton beams, or neutron beams to destroy cancer cells or keep them from reproducing.

**Testosterone**—The primary sex hormone in males, secreted by the testes, which stimulates the development of male sex organs, secondary sexual traits, and sperm. *See also* Androgen, Hormones.

**Testicles (Testes)**—The male sex organs located in the scrotum, which produce sperm and the hormone testosterone.

# Resources

## General

### Online

It is not difficult to find information about prostate cancer on the Internet. The fact is, there is too much information there for anyone to plow through! If one searches on Google for the following strings of words (with the quotes, which helps find specific phrases)—"prostate cancer" "side effects" "hormone therapy"—you will find *tens of millions* of hits. So how does one decide what is reliable, and what is not?!

Trustworthy sites are not necessarily embellished with music, animation, and videos. Sites with those fancy features are often the property of a commercial operation, which is trying to sell a product. Reliable sites indicate who owns them. The most reliable websites are not necessarily the most fancy ones.

If a site promotes a specific product for cancer treatment, it is wise to scroll to the bottom and look for small-print disclaimers. The owners of the site often display those disclaimers to state what their product is truly capable of doing. So, for example, the site might suggest that some herbal product is a "better way to fight prostate cancer," but then have a disclaimer saying that the information above is not really meant as an alternative treatment for cancer patients and is only posted for "educational purposes." The disclaimer is an effort to keep the owners out of legal trouble. Typically, it is better to trust these disclaimers than all of the text that comes before them.

Although there are exceptions to the following principles, websites with an extensive list of personal testimonials endorsing a particular cancer treatment should be viewed as suspect. The problem is that such testimonials are invariably biased, presenting a one-sided, typically positive, view of the topic. If a novel treatment failed to work, those individuals who did not benefit rarely provide testimonials As a general rule, competent and responsible websites do not rely on testimonials to justify the materials or information they offer.

In a recent analysis of otherwise reliable websites for information on ADT*, many websites owned by major nonprofit organizations were not up-to-date, even though they had a time stamp stating when they had last been updated. One website did stand out as having comprehensive current information: www.USTOO.org

## Support Groups

For gay men with prostate cancer: health.groups.yahoo.com/group/prostate-cancerandgaymen/

## Gynecomastia

Garments and compression shirts:
www.gynecomastiagarments.com
www.underarmour.com

## Benefits of Exercise

www.youtube.com/watch?v=aUaInS6HIGo

## Dietary Reference Intakes

Canada: www.hc-sc.gc.ca/fn-an/food-guide-aliment/index-eng.php.
United States: fnic.nal.usda.gov/dietary-guidance/dietary-reference-intakes

## Erotic Material

### Online

www.sexuality.org/
www.yourtango.com/2007282/passion-in-print.html
www.goaskalice.columbia.edu/1937.html
eroticaforwomen.com/
www.lovedreamer.com/ (products and info)

### Books

*Seductions: Tales of Erotic Persuasions, Erotic Interludes: Tales Told by Women* and *The Erotic Edge* by Lonnie Barbach, PhD. Dr. Barbach is a clinical psychologist who specializes in couples' therapy. The focus of her writing

---

*Ogah I, Wassersug RJ. How reliable are "reputable sources" for medical information on the Internet? The case of hormonal therapy to treat prostate cancer. *Urol Oncol.* 2012. 31(8):1546–1552

is on helping couples maintain healthy sex lives. The first two books listed here are mostly written for female audiences. The *Erotic Edge* was written for couples by couples and we recommend this book in particular for couples to read to each other as a way to stimulate sexual appetite.

*My Secret Garden, Forbidden Flowers and Women on Top* by Nancy Friday. Friday's books are mostly based on women's sexual fantasies but may still provide stimulating content for couples. These books document erotic stories that entertain a range of topics including sexual fantasies, relationships, jealousy, envy, feminism, BDSM, and beauty.

*Loving Sex: The Book of Joy and Passion* and *Real Sex for Real Women: Intimacy, Pleasure, and Sexual Well-Being* by Dr. Laura Berman. Dr. Berman is a sex educator and relationship specialist. Her books include provocative but also tasteful pictures as well as lots of resources about sexual positions, tips for arousal and orgasm, ideas about seduction, suggestions for stimulating fantasies, and tips for expanding your sexual repertoire. Exploring a book like this can provide a common ground for discussion and exploration with your partner.

## Distress, Relaxation, Coping, and Mindfulness

*Full Catastrophe Living* by Jon Kabat-Zinn. This book provides a thorough overview of mindfulness and its application to health and illness.

*Mindfulness-Based Cancer Recovery: A Step-by-Step MBSR Approach to Help You Cope with Treatment and Reclaim Your Life* by Linda Carlson and Michael Speca. This book covers an 8-week program that involves theory and practice designed specifically for cancer patients and their support persons.

*The Mindful Way through Depression* by J. Mark G. Williams, John D. Teasdale, Zindel V. Segal, and Jon Kabat-Zinn. This book provides an excellent introduction to mindfulness and it applications to psychological distress and/or depression.

*The Mindful Way through Anxiety: Break Free from Chronic Worry and Reclaim Your Life* by Susan M. Orsillo and Lizabeth Roemer. This book teaches mindfulness principles and skills to help in the management of chronic worry, anxiety and stress.

*The Anxiety and Phobia Workbook* by Edmund J. Bourne. This workbook is an excellent step-by-step self-help program based on cognitive-behavioral therapy that is highly effective in the treatment of anxiety disorders.

# Bibliography

## Introduction to ADT

Fujimoto N, Kubo T, Shinsaka H, Matsumoto M, et al. Duration of androgen deprivation therapy with maximum androgen blockade for localized prostate cancer. *BMC Urol.* 2011;11:7.

Hussain M, Tangen CM, Berry DL, Higano CS, et al. Intermittent versus continuous androgen deprivation in prostate cancer. *N Engl J Med.* 2013;368(14):1314–1325.

Lin YH, Chen CL, Hou CP, Chang PL, et al. A comparison of androgen deprivation therapy versus surgical castration for patients with advanced prostatic carcinoma. *Acta Pharmacol Sin.* 2011;32(4):537–542.

Walker LM, Tran S, Wassersug RJ, Thomas B, et al. Patients and partners lack knowledge of androgen deprivation therapy side effects. *Urol Oncol.* 2013;31(7):1098–1105.

Warde P, Mason M, Ding K, Kirkbride P, et al. Combined androgen deprivation therapy and radiation therapy for locally advanced prostate cancer: a randomized, phase 3 trial. *Lancet.* 2011;378(9809):2104–2111.

Wolff JM. Intermittent androgen deprivation in advanced prostate cancer: a review. *Aktuelle Urol.* 2012;43(2):115–120.

## Understanding the Physical Side Effects of ADT

Alibhai SM, Breunis H, Timilshina N, Johnston C, et al. Impact of androgen-deprivation therapy on physical function and quality of life in men with nonmetastatic prostate cancer. *J Clin Oncol.* 2010;28(34):5038–4505.

Elliot SE, Latini DM, Walker LM, Robinson JW, et al. Androgen deprivation therapy for prostate cancer: recommendations to improve quality of life. *J Sex Med.* 2010;7(9):2996–3010.

Grunfeld EA, Halliday A, Martin P, Drudge-Coates L. Andropause syndrome in men treated for metastatic prostate cancer: a qualitative study of the impact of symptoms. *Cancer Nurs.* 2012;35(1):63–69.

Saylor PJ, Smith MR. Adverse effects of androgen deprivation therapy: defining the problem and promoting health among men with prostate cancer. *J Natl Compr Canc Netw.* 2010;8(2):211–223.

## Cardiovascular and Diabetic Risk

Alibhai SM. Cardiovascular toxicity of androgen deprivation therapy: a new door opens. *J Clin Oncol.* 2011;29(26):3500–3502.

Aversa A, Francomano D, Lenzi A. Cardiometabolic complications after androgen deprivation therapy in a man with prostate cancer: effects of 3 years intermittent testosterone supplementation. *Front Endocrinol (Lausanne).* 2012;3:17.

Keating NL, Liu PH, O'Malley AJ, Freedland SJ, et al. Androgen-deprivation therapy and diabetes control among diabetic men with prostate cancer. *Eur Urol.* 2014;64(5):816–824.

Martín-Merino E, Johansson S, Morris T, García Rodríguez LA. Androgen deprivation therapy and the risk of coronary heart disease and heart failure in patients with prostate cancer: a nested case-control study in UK primary care. *Drug Saf.* 2011;34(11):1061–1077.

Mohamedali HZ, Alibhai SMH. Does androgen deprivation therapy increase diabetes risk? *Diabetes Manage.* 2011;1(6):551–553.

Nguyen PL, Je Y, Schutz FA, Hoffman KE, et al. Association of androgen deprivation therapy with cardiovascular death in patients with prostate cancer: a meta-analysis of randomized trials. *JAMA.* 2011;306(21):2359–2366.

Nobes JP, Langley SE, Klopper T, Russell-Jones D, et al. A prospective, randomized pilot study evaluating the effects of metformin and lifestyle intervention on patients with prostate cancer receiving androgen deprivation therapy. *BJU Int.* 2012;109(10):1495–1502.

Spratt DE, Zhang C, Zumsteg ZS, Pei X, et al. Metformin and prostate cancer: reduced development of castration-resistant disease and prostate cancer mortality. *Eur Urol.* 2013;63(4):709–716.

Timilshina N, Hussain S, Breunis H, Alibhai SM. Predictors of hemoglobin decline in nonmetastatic prostate cancer patients on androgen deprivation therapy: a matched cohort study. *Support Care Cancer.* 2011;19(11):1815–1821.

## Hot Flashes

Engstrom CA. Hot flashes in prostate cancer: state of the science. *Am J Mens Health.* 2008;2(2):122–132.

Frisk J. Managing hot flushes in men after prostate cancer: a systematic review. *Maturitas.* 2010;65(1):15–22.

Moraska AR, Atherton PJ, Szydlo DW, Barton DL, et al. Gabapentin for the management of hot flashes in prostate cancer survivors: a longitudinal continuation study-NCCTG trial N00CB. *J Support Oncol.* 2010;8(3):128–132.


## Bone Health

Alibhai SM, Yun L, Cheung AM, Paszat L. Screening for osteoporosis in men receiving androgen deprivation therapy. *JAMA.* 2012;307(3):255–256.

Beebe-Dimmer JL, Cetin K, Shahinian V, Morgenstern H, et al. Timing of androgen deprivation therapy use and fracture risk among elderly men with prostate cancer in the United States. *Pharmacoepidemiol Drug Saf.* 2012;21(1):70–78.

Lee CE, Leslie WD, Czaykowski P, Gingerich J, et al. A comprehensive bone-health management approach for men with prostate cancer receiving androgen deprivation therapy. *Curr Oncol.* 2011;18(4):e163–72.

Serpa Neto A, Tobias-Machado M, Esteves MA, Senra MD. Bisphosphonate therapy in patients under androgen deprivation therapy for prostate cancer: a systematic review and meta-analysis. *Prostate Cancer Prostatic Dis.* 2012;15(1):36–44.


## Weight Gain

Timilshina N, Breunis H, Alibhai SM. Impact of androgen deprivation therapy on weight gain differs by age in men with nonmetastatic prostate cancer. *J Urol.* 2012;188(6):2183–2188.


## Fatigue

Langston B, Armes J, Levy A, Tidey E, et al. The prevalence and severity of fatigue in men with prostate cancer: a systematic review of the literature. *Support Care Cancer.* 2013;21(6):1761–1771.


## Exercise Recommendations for Patients on ADT

Bolam KA, Galvão DA, Spry N, Newton RU, et al. AST-induced bone loss in men with prostate cancer: exercise as a potential countermeasure. *Prostate Cancer Prostatic Dis.* 2012;15(4):329–338.

Cormie P, Newton RU, Taaffe DR, Spry N, et al. Exercise maintains sexual activity in men undergoing androgen suppression for prostate cancer: a randomized controlled trial. *Prostate Cancer Prostatic Dis.* 2012;16(2):170–175.

Galvão DA, Taaffe DR, Spry N, Joseph D, et al. Acute versus chronic exposure to androgen suppression for prostate cancer: impact on the exercise response. *J Urol.* 2011;186(4):1291–1297.

Lee CE, Leslie WD, Lau YK. A pilot study of exercise in men with prostate cancer receiving androgen deprivation therapy. *BMC Cancer.* 2012;12:103.

Murphy R, Wassersug RJ, Dechman G. The role of exercise in managing the adverse effects of androgen deprivation therapy in men with prostate cancer. *Physical Therapy Reviews.* 2011;16(4):269–277.

Newton RU, Taaffe DR, Spry N, Cormie P, et al. Can exercise ameliorate treatment toxicity during the initial phase of testosterone deprivation in prostate cancer patients? Is this more effective than delayed rehabilitation? *BMC Cancer.* 2012;12:432.

Thorsen L, Nilsen TS, Raastad T, Courneya KS, et al. A randomized controlled trial on the effectiveness of strength training on clinical and muscle cellular outcomes in patients with prostate cancer during androgen deprivation therapy: rationale and design. *BMC Cancer.* 2012;12:123.

Winters-Stone KM, Schwartz A, Nail LM. A review of exercise interventions to improve bone health in adult cancer survivors. *J Cancer Surviv.* 2010:4(3):187–201.

## Healthy Eating and ADT

Brasky TM, Darke AK, Song X, Tangen CM, et al. Plasma phospholipid fatty acids and prostate cancer risk in the SELECT trial. *J Natl Cancer Inst.* 2013;105(15):1015–1016.

Freedland SJ, Aronson WJ. Dietary intervention strategies to modulate prostate cancer risk and prognosis. *Curr Opin Urol.* 2009;19(3):263–267.

Hardin J, Cheng I, Witte JS. Impact of consumption of vegetable, fruit, grain, and high glycemic index foods on aggressive prostate cancer risk. *Nutr Cancer.* 2011;63(6):860–872.

Harvard University Health Services. 2004. Calcium content of common foods in common portions. Available at huhs.harvard.edu/assets/File/OurServices/Service_Nutrition_CalciumContentOfCommonFoods.pdf; accessed on January 2014.

Health Canada. 2007. What is a food guide serving of meat and alternatives? Available at www.hcsc.gc.ca/fn-an/food-guide-aliment/choose-choix/meat-viande/serving-portion-eng.php; accessed January 2014.

Health Canada. *Canadian Guidelines for Body Weight Classification in Adults.* Ottawa, ON: Minister of Public Works and Government Services Canada; 2003.

Hori S, Butler E, McLoughlin J. Prostate cancer and diet: food for thought? *BJU Int.* 2011;107(9):1348–1359.

Nimptsch K, Kenfield S, Jensen MK, Stampfer MJ, et al. Dietary glycemic index, glycemic load, insulin index, fiber and whole-grain intake in relation to risk of prostate cancer. *Cancer Causes Control.* 2011;22(1):51–61.

Office of Dietary Supplements. 2013. Dietary supplement fact sheet: calcium. National Institutes of Health. Available at ods.od.nih.gov/factsheets/ Calcium-HealthProfessional/; accessed on January 2014.

Trachtenberg J, Fleshner N, Currie KL, Santa Mina D, et al. *Challenging Prostate Cancer: Nutrition, Exercise, and You.* Toronto, ON: The Prostate Centre; 2008.

## Effects on Mood and Emotional Well-Being

Casey RG, Corcoran NM, Goldenberg SL. Quality-of-life issues in men undergoing androgen deprivation therapy: a review. *Asian J Androl.* 2012; 14(2):226–231.

Chipperfield K, Fletcher J, Millar J, Brooker J, et al. Predictors of depression, anxiety, and quality of life in patients with prostate cancer receiving androgen deprivation therapy. *Psychooncology.* 2013; 22(10):2169–2176.

Kan C, Silva N, Golden SH, Rajala U, et al. A systematic review and meta-analysis of the association between depression and insulin resistance. *Diabetes Care.* 2013;36(2):480–489.

Kornblith AB, Herr HW, Ofman US, Scher HI, et al. Quality of life of patients with prostate cancer and their spouses. The value of a database in clinical care. *Cancer.* 1994;73(11):2791–2802.

Wikman A, Wardle J, Steptoe A. Quality of life and affective well-being in middle-aged and older people with chronic medical illnesses: a cross-sectional population-based study. *PLoS One.* 2011;6(4):e18952.

## Effects on Cognition

Alibhai SM, Mohamedali HZ. Cardiac and cognitive effects of androgen deprivation therapy: Are they real? *Curr Oncol.* 2010;17(suppl 2):S55–S64.

Alibhai SM, Breunis H, Timilshina N, Marzouk S, et al. Impact of androgen-deprivation therapy on cognitive function in men with nonmetastatic prostate cancer. *J Clin Oncol.* 2010;28(34):5030–5037.

Jamadar RJ, Winters MJ, Maki PM. Cognitive changes associated with ADT: a review of the literature. *Asian J Androl.* 2012;14(2):232–238.

Mohile SG, Lacy M, Rodin M, Bylow K, et al. Cognitive effects of androgen deprivation therapy in an older cohort of men with prostate cancer. *Crit Rev Oncol Hematol.* 2010;75(2):152–159.

Nelson CJ, Lee JS, Gamboa MC, Roth AJ. Cognitive effects of hormone therapy in men with prostate cancer: a review. *Cancer.* 2008;113(5):1097–1106.

Wu LM, Diefenbach MA, Gordon WA, Cantor JB, et al. Cognitive problems in patients on androgen deprivation therapy: a qualitative pilot study. *Urol Oncol.* 2013;31(8):1533–1538.

## Effects on Sexuality

Higano CS. Sexuality and intimacy after definitive treatment and subsequent androgen deprivation therapy for prostate cancer. *J Clin Oncol.* 2012;30(30):3720–3725.

Park KK, Lee SH, Chung BH. The effects of long-term androgen deprivation therapy on penile length in patients with prostate cancer: a single-center, prospective, open-label, observational study. *J Sex Med.* 2011;8(11):3214–3219.

Walker LM, Hampton AJ, Wassersug RJ, Thomas BC, et al. Androgen deprivation therapy and maintenance of intimacy: a randomized controlled pilot study of an educational intervention for patients and their partners. *Contemp Clin Trials.* 2013;34(2):227–231.

Warkentin KM, Gray RE, Wassersug RJ. Restoration of satisfying sex for a castrated cancer patient with complete impotence: a case study. *J Sex Marital Ther.* 2006;32(5):389–399.

Wassersug RJ, Gray R. The health and well-being of prostate cancer patients and male-to-female transsexuals on androgen deprivation therapy: a qualitative study with comments on expectations and estrogen. *Psychol Health Med.* 2011;16(1):39–52.

Wibowo E, Schellhammer P, Wassersug RJ. Role of estrogen in normal male function: clinical implications for patients with prostate cancer on androgen deprivation therapy. *J Urol.* 2011;185(1):17–23.

## Effects on Intimate Relationships

Navon L, Morag A. Advanced prostate cancer patients' ways of coping with the hormonal therapy's effect on the body, sexuality, and spousal ties. *Qual Health Res.* 2003;13(10):1378–1392.

Walker LM, Robinson JW. The unique needs of couples experiencing androgen deprivation therapy for prostate cancer. *J Sex Marital Ther.* 2010;36(2):154–165.

Walker LM, Robinson JW. A description of heterosexual couples' sexual adjustment to androgen deprivation therapy for prostate cancer. *Psychooncology.* 2011;20(8):880–888.

# Acknowledgments

This book would not have been possible without the contributions of the ADT Working Group, a collection of approximately twenty people, including PhDs, MDs, nurses, and graduate students, who work with and are dedicated to helping prostate cancer patients recognize and manage the side effects of their treatments. Established in 2008, the members of the ADT Working Group have been instrumental in helping us to research, write, field test, edit, and revise this book. The authors and many contributors to this book are a part of the ADT Working Group.

We would also like to acknowledge the following people for their contributions:

Deborah McLeod who is a founding member and driving force of the ADT Working Group.

Daniel Santa Mina and Andrew Matthew for their contributions to the development and writing of the chapter on exercise (as well, Andrew provided feedback and editorial revisions on the entire ADT book). Special thanks to Nicole Culos-Reed for reviewing the chapter on exercise.

Andrew Matthew and Kristen Currie for their contributions to the chapter on healthy eating. Special thanks to Cheri Van Patten for reviewing that chapter, as well as updating and adapting its content for our U.S. audience.

The authors praise Kirsten Kukula as *the* definitive editor of this volume. Kirsten not only edited multiple drafts of the manuscripts, but undertook key literature searches that contributed materially to every chapter in this book. We thank her profusely for tightening our writing and reducing redundancies in the text. Every page has profited from her clarity of thought and her comprehensive overview of the project. Erik Wibowo took on the challenging task of helping with the final copy editing of the book. We thank them both for their technical help.

Several physicians involved in the care of prostate cancer patients on ADT for their critical review of the book, including Stacy Elliott, Shabbir Alibhai, Dean Ruether, Derek Wilke, and Peter Black.

The ADT Working Group has received financial support from a variety of sources. The initial meeting of the group in 2008 was supported by grants from the Nova Scotia Health Research Foundation, the Dalhousie Cancer Research Program (now the Beatrice Hunter Cancer Research Institute), and a private donation from Lori Wood, MD.

Development and assessment of an earlier edition of this book was supported by a grant from the Canadian Institutes of Health Research (Richard Wassersug and John Robinson, co-principal investigators). Lauren Walker's research in the development and assessment of the revised edition was supported by a Canadian Male Sexual Health Council Grant (John Robinson, PI), Social Sciences and Humanities Council of Canada Scholarship (Lauren Walker), Alberta Innovates–Health Solutions Scholarship (Lauren Walker), and the Program for Undergraduate Research Experience Award, University of Calgary (Linette Lawlor).

All of the associations in Vancouver for the first author were made possible by S. Larry Goldenberg, MD, who supported Wassersug's commitment to developing supportive care resources for prostate cancer patients and their families. Wassersug would, in addition, like to thank the Australian Research Centre in Sex, Health and Society for providing him a research home in the Southern hemisphere, and his colleagues down under that share his interests in helping prostate cancer patients recover from the side effects of their cancer treatments.

We are pleased to acknowledge, in alphabetical order, the pharmaceutical companies that manufacture and market medications used in treating prostate cancer, and have supported this work. We extend special thanks to Peter Black for bringing this project to the attention of all those companies. Their broad support attests to the companies' commitment to meet the needs of prostate cancer patients dealing with the consequences of ADT.

AbbVie
Amgen
AstellasPharmaCanada, Inc.
AstraZeneca Canada, Inc.

Ferring, Inc.
Johnson & Johnson Shared Services (Janssen Biotech, Inc.)
Sanofi Canada

Several institutions deserve special mention for the long-term support
that they have provided to the ADT Working Group:
- Dalhousie University, Capital Health and the Nova Scotia Cancer Centre in
  Halifax, Nova Scotia
- Tom Baker Cancer Centre, University of Calgary and  Prostate Cancer
  Center in Calgary, Alberta
- Vancouver General Hospital, Vancouver Prostate Centre, Bristish Columbia
  Cancer Agency and the University of British Columbia in Vancouver,
  British Columbia
- Princes Margaret Cancer Center in Toronto, Ontario.

# Index

# About the Authors

**Richard J. Wassersug, PhD,** is a research scientist who earned his doctoral degree in evolutionary biology from the University of Chicago. He then spent most of his career studying the biology of amphibians and teaching anatomy in the medical school at Dalhousie University in Halifax, Nova Scotia. At the age of 52, he was diagnosed with prostate cancer and has since been receiving multiple treatments for the disease. After beginning androgen deprivation therapy, he redirected his research to study the psychology of androgen deprivation in various populations. Richard is now an Adjunct Professor in the Department of Urologic Sciences at the University of British Columbia and Co-Lead of the Vancouver Prostate Centre's new Prostate Cancer Supportive Care Program.

**Lauren M. Walker, PhD,** received her doctorate in clinical psychology, and is a clinical fellow in the Department of Oncology at the University of Calgary and the Tom Baker Cancer Centre, Calgary, Alberta. She completed her dissertation research evaluating a patient education initiative for preparing prostate cancer patients (and their partners) starting androgen deprivation therapy. She works clinically with couples, helping them adapt to the sexual implications of cancer treatments. She is an active researcher, who has contributed several key articles to the scientific literature on the psychosocial adaptation to androgen deprivation therapy.

**John W. Robinson, PhD, R Psych,** has been a clinical psychologist and a member of the Genital Urinary Program at the Tom Baker Cancer Centre in Calgary, Alberta, since 1986. He concurrently provides clinical service and develops new ways to ease the psychological burden of cancer on not just patients but also their loved ones. He has appointments in both oncology and clinical psychology at the University of Calgary, where he teaches and carries on an active research program.

# About the Contributors

**Kristen L. Currie, MA, CCRP**, graduated in 2002 from Queen's University, in Kingston, Ontario, with concurrent degrees in life science, and physical and health education. She then completed a master's degree in 2005 in kinesiology (health psychology) at York University, in Toronto, Ontario. She has researched the nutrition behavior of men at risk of onset or recurrence of prostate cancer, and currently manages the Prostate Cancer Rehabilitation Clinic at Princess Margaret Cancer Centre in Toronto, Ontario.

**Kirsten C. Kukula, BSc**, holds a combined honors degree in biology and sociology from Dalhousie University. She works as a research assistant at Dalhousie University and the Capital Health District Authority, mainly on projects in the area of psychosocial oncology. Her areas of interest include the social determinants of health, sexuality, and medicine.

**Linette Lawlor-Savage, MSc**, is completing doctoral studies in clinical psychology at the University of Calgary. Her primary interest areas are neuropsychology and psychosocial oncology. Her current research utilizes behavioral and neuroimaging methods to investigate cognitive functioning (e.g., loss and recovery of abilities such as memory, thinking speed, and decision making) in healthy aging adults and in cancer survivors.

**Andrew Matthew, PhD, C Psych**, is a senior staff psychologist at the Princess Margaret Cancer Hospital, in Toronto, Ontario, where he is a clinician-investigator in the Department of Surgery, Division of Urology, and a member of the Department of Psychosocial Oncology and Palliative Care. He is also an assistant professor in the Faculty of Medicine, University of Toronto, Departments of Surgery and Psychiatry.

**Deborah McLeod, RN, PhD,** is a clinician scientist in nursing with the Queen Elizabeth II Cancer Care Program, in Halifax, Nova Scotia. She is a clinical member of the psychosocial oncology team, providing individual, couples, and family therapy. She conducts research with couples that are coping with cancer, with a focus on communication and sexuality.

**Daniel Santa Mina, CEP, PhD,** completed his doctoral studies at York University examining the psychosocial and physiological effects of exercise in men with prostate cancer. He is a Certified Exercise Physiologist with the Canadian Society for Exercise Physiology and holds certification as a Cancer Exercise Specialist from the Rocky Mountain Cancer Rehabilitation Institute, in Greeley, Colorado. Dr. Santa Mina is currently a Postdoctoral Fellow at the Prostate Centre in the Princess Margaret Cancer Centre, and the Program Head of Kinesiology at the University of Guelph-Humber, in Toronto, Ontario.

**Cheri Van Patten, RD, MSc,** is a registered dietitian with over 17 years of combined clinical and research experience in prostate cancer at the British Columbia Cancer Agency in Vancouver. Her areas of expertise and publications have included diet, body weight, obesity, exercise, and dietary supplements, and their impact on quality of life and risk of recurrence in cancer survivors.